PRAISE FOR PETE EGOSCUE AND PAIN FREE

"Shows how we can break the circuit of pain and naturally heal one of the most significant disabilities of our times."
—Deepak Chopra, author of *The Path of Love* and *The Seven Spiritual Laws of Success*

"Born from the genius of Pete Egoscue, the simple and effective routines in *Pain Free* are the cutting edge of physical therapy."
—Anthony Robbins, author of *Awaken the Giant Within* and *Unlimited Power*

"Pete Egoscue teaches you practical, powerful 'motioncises'—motion exercises that will become your own best exercise therapist."
—Harold Bloomfield, M.D., author of *How to Heal Depression*

Also by Pete Egoscue with Roger Gittines

PAIN FREE
PAIN FREE FOR WOMEN

BANTAM BOOKS
New York   Toronto   London
Sydney   Auckland

PAIN FREE
AT YOUR PC

Pete Egoscue

with

Roger Gittines

PAIN FREE AT YOUR PC
A Bantam Book / November 1999

BOOK DESIGN BY GLEN M. EDELSTEIN

Library of Congress Cataloging-in-Publication Data
Egoscue, Pete
    Pain free at your PC / Pete Egoscue, with Roger Gittines. p. cm.
Includes index.
ISBN 978-0-553-38052-1
1. Microcomputers—Health aspects.   2. Pain—Prevention.
I. Gittines, Roger.   II. Title.
RC95.V53E36 1999
613.6'2—dc21   99-26664
                                                CIP

Published simultaneously in the United States and Canada

PRINTED IN THE UNITED STATES OF AMERICA

CONTENTS

As for all my books, I provide a disclaimer with a difference. Instead of the usual "The following material is not intended as a substitute for the advice of a physician," followed by a recommendation that you consult a doctor before following the program that's being offered and a disclaimer of legal responsibility should there be adverse consequences, I take another approach. Don't read this book if you feel you need the protection of a disclaimer and its counsel. I'm serious. Health care must start with personal responsibility. This vital role should not be delegated to any expert. Yours is the ultimate judgment. Any disclaimer that suggests otherwise does a great disservice.

List of Illustrations

Chapter 3

Chapter 4

Chapter 9

Chapter 11

Chapter 12

Chapter 13

Acknowledgments

I feel like I'm rounding up the usual suspects. The first is Roger Gittines, my coauthor. A beautiful friendship continues, as well as a solid partnership that has now yielded three books—with more to follow. Thanks again to Brian Bradley, the Egoscue Method Clinic director, and Erica Lusk, video therapy director, for being such good functional models and good sports. Therapists Liba, Paul, and Jamie provided valuable assistance.

Artist Wendy Wray's drawings give new meaning to the old line "Seeing is believing." Photographer Scott Crain came through for us with high-quality work under tight deadline pressure. Robin Michaelson, our editor, made life pain free, and her boss Irwyn Applebaum gave us a second chance. He runs a first-class operation.

PAIN FREE AT YOUR PC

1

THE PC—FROM PAINFUL TO PAIN FREE

"The true source of chronic musculoskeletal pain is rarely the site of the pain. . . . If your wrist hurts while you are pointing and clicking with a mouse, the pain probably has nothing to do with the device."

"It's a deal. Let's shake on it."

"I can't, my wrist hurts."

"Hah! I told you that was going to happen."

"I know, but my career's golden. I'm on the cutting edge."

"Cutting edge? High-tech hell is more like it."

"I'm going to try a wrist splint. I've got a shinbone of a musk ox I can use."

"Try getting another job. Your wrist is always going to hurt. Humans weren't designed to swing a hammer all day. Your basic rock was good enough."

Musk ox? Hammer? A quick visit to a Pleistocene valley startup? Sorry for the cheap trick, but it probably worked. I know *you* saw right through me, but many other readers thought I was referring to that dreaded public health menace, the personal computer—wrecker of wrists, despoiler of eyesight, inflamer of elbows, cricker of necks, and begetter of headaches.

And now I am in more trouble because it may seem like I'm being unsympathetic to people experiencing agonizing pain. But on that charge, as someone who's spent almost every day of nearly the last thirty years helping those suffering from chronic musculoskeletal pain, I plead not guilty. Millions of men, women, and children are hurting. The sleepless nights are real, as is the inability to tie shoelaces and the struggle to surmount the wall of pain that stands in the way of pointing and clicking with a mouse or tapping the space bar of a keyboard with a thumb. Likewise, the stiff necks and nauseating headaches destroy productivity and any sense of a job well done.

No, I'm deeply sympathetic to those in chronic pain. I've been there myself, and my search for a cure to relieve my pain led to the formulation of a therapeutic method, the Egoscue Method, that is now known worldwide as a remarkably successful alternative to drastic drug and surgical treatments or gimmicky "ergonomic" solutions that do more harm than good.

My point about the PC and the hammer is this: Just as it would be wrong to blame the hammer for the aches and pains that beset workers from the era of the caveman to the cabinetmaker, the coal miner to the carpenter, it's a mistake to think that the personal computer is responsible for the variety of conditions that are being labeled "computer pain syndrome."

The term is as inapt as *hammer pain syndrome, fountain pen pain syndrome,* or *microscope pain syndrome.* These are tools, not diseases. We've flourished as toolmakers and tool users—our tools are blameless. Certainly, accidents happen on the job. Safety must always be a priority, although it frequently isn't. But to treat a tool—any tool, high tech or low—as the source of an epidemic is something new and profoundly disturbing.

Whatever pain you may be feeling, it is not caused by your PC. And it cannot be cured by reinventing the PC or the way you use it. There is a remedy, though, and that's what this book is all about.

Pain Free at Your PC challenges conventional wisdom with what I regard to be the most persuasive and conclusive body of evidence—the human body. Being pain free at your PC is as natural and attainable as a pain-free night's sleep or a pain-free day of hard work. Our hands and wrists are inherently strong enough to operate a keyboard and a mouse for hours on end. Human necks, heads, and eyes can take the stress and strain too.

So what's the problem? Why is the federal government describing repetitive stress injuries (RSIs) as a workplace "epidemic"?

Why is the incidence of carpal tunnel syndrome (CTS) and other forms of chronic pain associated with computer use rising dramatically?

Why are we quick to blame this valuable new tool?

The answer is that a search for the *cause* of computer-related pain has veered off course and locked onto the *effect* instead. Let me filter this predicament through an observation I made early in my career as a therapist: **The true source of chronic musculoskeletal pain is rarely the site of the pain.** That means if your wrist hurts while you are pointing and clicking with a mouse, the pain probably has nothing to do with the device, and everything to do with muscular weakness, skeletal misalignment, and structural (joint) instability elsewhere in the body. Those conditions can be reversed without drastic measures—*and you can do it yourself.*

I've also learned that muscular weakness, skeletal misalignment, and structural instability usually *precede* the onset of pain that is attributed to accidents, overuse, or aging. That's right, precede. And that means we're ignoring the real cause of the pain when we tinker with the PC or the mouse, replace the chair, brace the wrist, or surgically remove the transverse carpal ligament (the usual CTS surgical procedure). The symptoms may abate temporarily because peripheral conditions have changed, but the pain usually returns or shifts to another spot. We're better off retracing our steps to correct—here's the chorus again—muscular weakness, skeletal misalignment, and structural instability. Just call them *dysfunctions* to save time.

Remembering to Forget

It's easy to draw the wrong conclusion about PCs when cause and effect get jumbled around. The PC seems to be placing an inordinate demand on our physical functions by asking us to move our fingers, hands, wrists, and arms again and again. And that's true. But it's only because we come to the PC expecting to use muscles and joints that were drained of much of their strength and flexibility long before Bill Gates made his first billion dollars. As modern specialists, we are now using special tools under special conditions. In itself that's no problem. Amnesia is the problem. We forget that our bodies evolved in service to the all-purpose, multifaceted work and lifestyles of a species of magnificent generalists. By remembering where we came from and who we are, we can forget the pain.

The musculoskeletal system is a virtual historical textbook chronicling the varied and demanding everyday movements required of humankind for millions of years. Look at it. Look at yourself. The erect spine and the rugged shoulders, the solid hips and the hard-driving knees, the sturdy ankles, tough feet, and clever hands are all chapters of a success story about creatures who could not keep still.

As an exercise therapist, when I "read" the text, I see an integrated, balanced unit of muscles and joints that must be fed or refueled *in its entirety* by motion. Although the world has changed, the musculoskeletal system remains the same—still magnificent, still a generalist after all those years. Our specialized work, however, restricts and limits motion to the relatively few muscles and joints that are directly involved. Even our recreational activity is specialized. Relatively few muscles work and play; all the rest languish.

Surgery, drugs, and ergonomic redesign do not address this fundamental source of chronic musculoskeletal pain.

Hardworking fingers, wrists, and hands cannot be isolated from nonworking (or minimally working) hips, knees, ankles, and their supporting musculature without painful consequences. The necessary mechanical and muscular interaction is lost. As a result, our integrated bodies are *disintegrating* and being deconditioned—not by the PC but by the TV, the CD, the RV, and all the other "A to E-Z" accoutrements of modern living. Our bodies are in trouble before we even sit down at the computer keyboard. Overall lack of motion and highly restricted specialized motion are the culprits. I'll explain the phenomenon in the remainder of this chapter and in chapters 2 and 3. After addressing the whys, the book will focus on what—what you can do about it quickly and easily.

And that's both good and bad news. Good because there is a solution; bad in that it requires a personal commitment to make small but significant changes in the way you live and work. Frankly, it's probably a bad idea to acknowledge this downside. Many people are turned off by the notion that they won't be able to buy good health just like any other product. Surgery, painkilling drugs, and products like ergonomic keyboards, wrist braces, and special desk chairs hold the promise of a quick fix. As dedicated consumers, we tend to believe we can purchase nearly anything that's needed ready-made and right off the shelf. Unfortunately, the human body doesn't work that way.

Did I use the word *unfortunately*? Actually, this is an entirely fortunate situation. Bones, joints, muscles, tendons, and ligaments maintain and sustain themselves on the go. All we have to do is *go* and keep going. The changes in your work and lifestyle that this book promotes are designed to take the stops out.

E-Therapy

As I do at my Egoscue Method Clinic in Del Mar, California, this book offers a program of "no sweat" E-cises—shorthand for Egoscue-cises, but the term could well be "Easy-cises." The body's musculoskeletal system doesn't require heavy workouts to function properly. That's why I refer to E-cises as "No Sweats," since you'll be able to do them in your office dressed in business clothes, and many can be performed sitting down with little interruption to your work routine.

These E-cises are culled from the hundreds I've devised from scratch based on a close study of human motion requirements. Many are also adapted from yoga positions, posture-enhancement routines, or classic therapeutic movements. Each one provides stimulation to specific muscle groups, joints, and functions that are not being used adequately or that are being abused by skeletal misalignment.

The results speak for themselves. In 1998 more than a thousand repetitive stress injury sufferers came to the clinic for treatment. In addition, I've worked with world-class professional and amateur athletes striving for peak performance, accident victims determined to recover, elderly people fighting to maintain their quality of life, and those with severe workplace injuries and disabilities who refuse to give up. We haven't used drugs or surgery. Our success rate is around 94 percent. The few disappointments came from a client's unwillingness or inability to commit to spending as little as twenty minutes a day doing specific E-cises.

The Common Cadence of Different Drummers

Most people who visit the clinic or take part in our home video therapy program have one thing in common—chronic pain. I assume the same is true for my readers. If not, and you're being proactive, you've also come to the right place. I'm glad you did. Pain or no pain, it's important to understand that almost all of us were born with the same musculoskeletal design. The difference—why one person has agonizing pain, a second some tightness, and a third no overt symptoms at all—is caused by what we do or don't do with that design. In that way everybody is, in fact, different: different jobs, different lifestyles, different hobbies, and different interests. At first those differences seem to make a consistent therapeutic response to chronic pain impossible. But the universal design of the body saves the day. Over the last twenty-five years, the E-cise programs that this book offers have been proven effective in helping people get back to using their body's musculoskeletal system in accordance with that basic design. They amount to tutorials. Weakened, disengaged muscles literally forget how and when to move according to design. The E-cises give them a quick refresher course.

You'll notice that in many cases the E-cises do not directly target the site of the pain symptom. The focus may be on the shoulders or hips rather than a sore neck or wrist. Why? Hit the "back button" on the browser and return to my first observation, a page or three ago: The body is so carefully balanced and functionally interrelated that the place where we feel the pain is usually a long way from its source. This is particularly true of the hands and wrists.

To see what I mean, clench your fist. Do it a couple of times. Clench and relax. Feel movement in your forearm, elbow, and shoulder? Good. That's where the prime muscular movers are located in order to keep the hands and wrists compact and flexible. The muscles themselves are elongated; their tendons are among the longest in the body. The arrangement allows for both a powerful grasp and fine joint articulation in the fingers. Otherwise, our hands would be crude and cumbersome.

The E-cises in *Pain Free at Your PC* reflect this principle of anatomy: The site of the pain and the source of the problem are often not the same. If that strikes you as repetitious, better get used to it. You'll read it several more times.

The immediate purpose of the E-cise program is to reengage and strengthen muscles that aren't being adequately sustained by your physical activities away from the PC. At the same time, they restore lost skeletal alignment that sets in when key functions are disrupted. It's pointless to "buff" muscles that are not doing their jobs properly or to struggle to reduce inflammation in the wrist when the source of the problem is the elbow or shoulder. Pain, stiffness, and swelling are symptoms. E-cises treat root causes and thereby eliminate both the symptom and the dysfunctions they generate. In addition they produce an increase in energy, strength, and your sense of well-being.

Since long before *Gray's Anatomy* was published in 1858, medical researchers have known that muscles lose strength and proper function when they are not used. It's pure supply and demand. The supply and effectiveness of muscle power grows in direct proportion to the demands we make on those muscles. In the pages ahead, I will point to the reasons why fewer and fewer muscles and the functions they support are being regularly used, and why there is a growing muscular-demand deficit. The E-cises in chapters 6 through 9 are intended to fill the gap and balance supply and demand.

Throughout this book I will challenge misconceptions about the way the body's muscles and joints work. One prevailing myth is that overuse or repetitive use of muscles and joints is dangerous. By now I hope you are beginning to realize that the opposite is the case. In almost every instance, underuse is central to the "Painful PC."

Underuse is happening head to toe. It's happening to computer users and concert pianists, football players and financiers; to the fit and flabby, to the young and old. Knees are blowing, hips are crumbling, lumbar disks are rupturing. For PC users, the front line, the primary hurting zone, involves the hands and wrists. Again, it's caused by underuse. The joints and muscles of this zone have been left to fend for themselves by allied muscles and joints that are supposed to be interactively supporting and assisting the job of finger flexing and extending, thumb waggling, gripping, grabbing, and stretching. Some muscles and joints are working like crazy, while others are in an it's-crazy-to-work mode.

By misdiagnosing this as overuse, the prescription then becomes one that is based on promoting underuse. Lock the wrist, back, or neck in a brace; stop using a keyboard; get a new job that doesn't require a computer. The effective remedy is use—proper use.

Another myth is that ergonomic gadgets can provide "workarounds" to patch the body's weak spots. These workarounds are actually masking dysfunctions and making the body weaker and more unstable. That's not what ergonomic experts intended, but that's what's happening.

And the third myth is that high technology supplants muscle power. A computer—the kind we use today, anyway—is a hand tool, and like any hand tool, be it a hammer or a pair of scissors, it makes specific demands on the body, far more than we realize. To respond to that demand, the musculoskeletal design must be intact and functional, which includes skeletal alignment, joint flexibility, and muscular strength. For most of us those requirements are not being met but can be with a little effort. That's our objective here.

My job is to help you achieve it. There's no reason that the sons and daughters of miners, millers, bridge-builders, and bricklayers should meet their match in the form of a computer keyboard, mouse, and video display terminal. Let's remember and renew our pain-free physical heritage as magnificent generalists, and leave the magnificent PC to evolve like any other useful tool.

MUSCLE2MATTERS

"For modern men and women, primary muscles from head to foot are disengaging. . . . There is stress, friction, and breakdown."

My work has given me enormous respect for the intricate yet fundamentally simple resilience of the human body. From spry old ladies to strapping young athletes and agile kids, I've closely examined the musculoskeletal system and how its rugged design allows us to function in direct response to the demands of harsh, unforgiving environments—even the harsh, unforgiving environment of a software programmer's cubicle at three o'clock in the morning.

Our earliest ancestors didn't go to work in cubicles—work came to them on all fours, in all four seasons, and from four points of the compass. The musculoskeletal system we inherited is proof of that. The body's arrangement of muscles, bones, joints, and nerves enables a hungry man to reach over his head to pluck ripe apples or to bend down to dig through the snow and into the earth for edible roots. He can run from danger, climb a tree, and throw a spear (and make the weapon with his own hands as well).

Did I say *he*? I may use the masculine pronoun from time to time, but *she* is just as capable. Male or female, our distant ancestors *embodied* lives of motion.

Consequently, there is no fixed limit on our stretching, bending, climbing, or running. The reason for that is the almost constant

---

PLANET GYM

Our ancestors "worked out" constantly. The issue wasn't staying in shape—they wanted to stay alive. The human body's musculoskeletal functions evolved in a motion-rich environment. No matter where they were—prairie, desert, mountains, seacoast—men and women were required by necessity to keep moving. The enemy was inactivity. Like sharks that constantly swim to breathe, we move to build and retain muscular and skeletal functions.

---

demand for motion that came humankind's way from an always-challenging environment. In short we were designed to do what we can do—move—and do it over and over again, depending only on individual strength and stamina. Simple fatigue and exhaustion, not pain or musculoskeletal damage, are the natural circuit breakers. We are designed to rest or go to sleep, and return to work—return to movement—refreshed *and* stronger.

Think about that. With time off to recharge, along with adequate food and water, our human apple-picker, root-grubber, or spear-thrower made the Energizer Bunny look like roadkill. Motion is the price we pay for muscle. The more we use muscles, the more they strengthen. So do the joints. Our *batteries* are designed to run up rather than run down. In terms of evolution, it is the adaptable who survive. This musculoskeletal amplitude is one of the mainstays of human adaptability. Without it we wouldn't have lasted for more than a few centuries. The first drought or plague of locusts would have done us in.

Luckily, though, we have a nearly flawless musculoskeletal system. Nearly. The flaw is that our environment is no longer harsh and unforgiving. We tamed it by eliminating most of the constant working motion. And before you shout hurrah, let me point out that that's what's causing your wrist to hurt or those other symptoms attributed to "computer pain syndrome." The correct term should be "environmental pain syndrome." If motion is the price of muscles, pain is the price of lack of motion *and* muscle. The computer is not guilty!

Home on the Range

Muscles don't need to be bulging and rippling and hamlike to be strong; true strength is a matter of tone, accessibility, and function. Are they fully capable of responding when you need them? The test is their ability to meet your requirements. It's not a matter of conquering Mount Everest. If you are a postal worker, can you walk your route without a struggle? If you are a pizza-delivery person, can you climb a steep set of stairs? If you are a researcher, can you operate a computer keyboard? If not, it doesn't matter who you are or what you do, without this readily available underlying muscle strength, your health is doomed to be weak.

Being pain free at your PC or any other tool is all about strength, motion, and health. It comes in one package.

A few pages earlier, I noted that we are designed to do what we can do, and do it over and over again. The reverse is true too—we cannot do what we cannot do. By that I mean we can't live upside down, fly under our own power, swivel our heads 360 degrees, survive without food, water, or oxygen, and so on. There are limits, rules, requirements. As a species, we have known this for several million years and have rarely violated the design limits of the body except by accident or sheer folly. In either of those events, the consequences are instantaneous and drastic. The offender either stops what he or she is doing or perishes.

Do you think there's a bit of evolutionary logic involved here? Seems likely to me.

By establishing what our bodies can't do, we form an instinctive awareness of our range of motion—what we can do. We know that we can stretch, bend at the waist and knees, rotate the torso to the left and right, grasp and release with the fingers and hands, and—well, you get the picture. A picture of motion. We start this process as infants. It's both no big deal, and a very big deal.

But this picture of motion (and muscle) is misleading because we feel it more than we see it; over time it's more a product of remembrance than reality. We remember that we can twist and turn and stretch, but when we do not frequently call on our muscles to perform those actions, they lose the ability to respond. Initially—perhaps years go by—this escapes our attention. Yet the memory of our full range of motion is there, and when we do call on it, confident of an instant response, the answer is pain.

Let me tell you why. The hitch with range of motion—ROM—is that it comes in two forms, design range of motion—DROM—and individual range of motion—IROM. Think of the first as what the body is capable of doing, and the second as what the individual actually does with his or her bones, joints, muscles, and nerves. There is an enormous disparity. For instance, many people hardly ever reach straight up over their heads. The function is there as part of DROM, but IROM is not utilizing it. Over time this function becomes increasingly inaccessible.

Almost all of us—there are very, very few exceptions accounted for by rare birth defects—started out with the same design range of motion once we got past infancy and toddlerhood. Aside from size and some minor bone surface variations, all the musculoskeletal parts are the same and operate in an identical manner. This forms the platform or foundation for the familiar functions like stretching and bending that I've been discussing. If you'll stand up, I will demonstrate what I mean.

DROM AND IROM

Design range of motion—DROM—is like the specs for a car's mechanical systems or any structural design. There are established parameters for muscular contraction and the articulation of joints. Bone size may vary from individual to individual, but the basic configuration and surface characteristics of all femurs (thigh bones), for instance, are the same. Almost everyone starts with the standard equipment package.

Individual range of motion—IROM—however, amounts to arbitrarily assuming that mechanical specs are totally elastic. Why bother replacing the passenger-side shock absorbers if no one sits on that side? Why not block half the radiator to warm the car faster in the winter? IROM does the same, albeit unconsciously, by favoring the right knee over the left, or freezing the shoulders in a rounded, stooped posture. These IROM alterations to the body's *mechanism* produce a net loss of strength, flexibility, and function.

Up? Good. Now sit down again, please.

What happened? Let me guess. You stood by using a hand to push off from the desk or arms of the chair. It's also likely that you leaned forward, bending at your waist and letting your head drop forward until gravity sort of tugged you out of the chair waiting for your knees to engage. And in the process most of your weight was transferred to one hip and leg.

These contortions are characteristic of human design range of motion in only one crude way. You got to your feet. You were able to access enough DROM—the platform—to improvise your way out of the chair by using individual range of motion—a variety of shortcuts and inventive ploys, like that business with your head. Don't feel bad. Many people do the same thing. Their knee joints are not engaging, but their hips are, which means that their head must act as a counterweight to open the knee joint wide enough to lock and bear weight and to move into semivertical alignment with the hips. The head is doing what weak knee and thigh muscles, thwarted by overly strong hip muscles, cannot.

It's very ingenious. The knee was not specifically designed to be bailed out by one's head, neck, and shoulders, but design range of motion allows for wide tolerances, another reason why we are so adaptable. But the repeated improvisation becomes a mixed-up pattern of a few healthy functions and dysfunctional aberrations. This is what I mean by individual range of motion, and why I am determined to help reestablish your *full design range of motion.*

DROM is there—you're just not using most of it.

I want you to be able to stand up without head fakes and hand tricks. Rising to one's feet, weight balanced equally between them, shoulders and head back, knees and hips in neutral—and look, Ma, no hands!—are the characteristics of a fully functional design range of motion. Without access to DROM, none of us can expect to swing a hammer or use a computer keyboard without pain.

Am I saying that the ability to stand up without these extra efforts has something to do with operating a computer keyboard?

You bet it does!

Power Struggle

By and large it is the nature of the environment that each of us inhabits that determines the attributes of our individual range of motion. Until roughly fifty or sixty years ago, the environment was sufficiently untamed that DROM and IROM coincided for most of us. Watch the actors in silent films rise from chairs, walk, and bend. They look strange, but it's not just primitive filmmaking techniques. Their postures are erect and their gait-pattern functions (the way they walk) are engaged, unlike modern men and women, who are exhibiting the symptoms of a slow-motion collapse of their musculoskeletal systems.

Collapse is a strong word, but I mean it. We are losing access to our design range of motion, and with it goes our pain-free birthright. It's not just aesthetics. A sexy slouch may be read as coolly sullen or sophisticated, but slumping shoulders and rounded hips are sending a message in loud and clear body language that something is wrong. Pain may or may not be present. The initial symptoms could be poor concentration, fatigue, or anxiety. It may take sitting at a computer for several hours doing research on a term paper or typing software code before a wrist starts getting stiff. Eventually, IROM and DROM will go to war.

The problem isn't that our bodies are frail or that the demands of operating a PC's keyboard and mouse are too strenuous. What's happening is that we've adopted a lifestyle that cannot automatically main-

TAKE A LOAD OFF

The mass-produced car, the modern office, power tools, and home labor-saving appliances were invented this century. Each of these breakthroughs replaced muscle power. Cars and offices meant that humans could sit down to travel and work, two activities formerly done mostly on foot. Power tools and home appliances mean that back, shoulder, and arm muscles aren't being used nearly as much. How are these muscles and joints stimulated? Very little. Consequently, they are not strong enough to carry out their primary responsibilities or to fully support other interrelated functions like typing or sitting up straight.

tain the health of our musculoskeletal system by keeping DROM and IROM reasonably compatible. Just as we work to master new software applications, we have to learn how to replace environmental stimulus ourselves. There are easy-to-use techniques for restoring and maintaining DROM that will prevent pain associated with computer use. I'll introduce them to you in chapters 6 through 9, but first I want to spend a little more time acquainting you with how the human body's hardware functions.

MUSCLE HEAD

Skeletal muscles tell the bones what to do.
Skeletal muscles come in pairs.
Skeletal muscles pull (contract) and relax, they don't push.
Skeletal muscles have assigned primary tasks.
Skeletal muscles never function in isolation.
Muscles constitute about 40 percent of the average person's body weight. Bones contribute another 20 percent.

Many people try to argue with me when I say that muscles tell the bones what to do. They contend that the brain, via nerves, calls the shots. And that's actually half right. The nerves transmit a signal, the muscle tissue contracts, and a bone moves. In due course the muscle's partner contracts and moves the bone back to where it started. The muscle is the middleman. It obeys the message—sometimes. When DROM and IROM are at odds, the message gets garbled, goes to the wrong bones, or is ignored.

This situation isn't a disease. It is a natural state. An inactive muscle loses its capacity to contract. An inefficient organism doesn't waste resources on unused functions. Hence the more inactivity, the more incapacity. Eventually, no matter how much a nerve demands a particular muscular response—move those fingers!—the muscles cannot obey.

That's when individual range of motion kicks in. IROM tries to keep the body moving in spite of muscular incapacity. When the

---

TWO JOBS, TWO MUSCLES

Skeletal muscles work in pairs: one flexing, the other extending. (Some do both, but only when they control more than one joint.) In both cases the muscles are contracting. A *flexor* muscle is pulling two bones toward each other. It then relaxes and an *extensor* pulls them away. Contract-relax-contract-relax. The best illustration of this action is your elbow. Tuck either the right or left elbow into your side. With the forearm held at a ninety-degree angle to start, without moving your elbow, bring your palm toward your shoulder—that's flexion. Move it back to the original position— that's extension. (Full extension would occur when the elbow joint is wide open and the arm is straight at your side.)

---

nerve's request to move muscle A is ignored, muscle B, C, or J will be recruited to assist. When I asked you to stand, and if you pushed off from the desk or chair with your hands, the muscles and joints of the hand, wrist, elbow, upper arms, shoulder, and upper back were augmenting or substituting for the muscles of the hips, thighs, and lower back.

This muscular *compensation,* to use the term I prefer, isn't all bad. Compensating muscles allow the body to deal with emergencies or to operate from an awkward position. They get the job done. Even so, doing it over and over again means that the bypassed muscles with the primary assignment get less and less stimulus. They weaken and disengage. The flexion-and-extension pairing is disrupted. There may be full flexion followed by a partial extension; like a hinge, the joint opens but doesn't fully close. The combinations and gradations are almost infinite. Try to imagine the chaos that goes on when several joints are behaving this way while they are attempting to function together. In that simple act of standing up that you did at my request, at least one or both hip joints were staying in flexion and not returning to neutral. Try it again right now.

Up? Look at your feet. If one or both are flared out, it is a symptom of your hip being held in flexion. What can't be seen easily is the contortions that the knees and ankles have undergone in reaction to the dysfunctional movement of the hips. Likewise, the lumbar vertebrae (the vertebrae of the lower back) weren't able to function properly. The effects run straight up the spine and influence how your shoulders, arms, wrists, and hands interact with a computer keyboard.

For modern men and women, primary muscles from head to foot are disengaging to an alarming degree. Secondary muscles are being recruited to do work that they are unsuited for. There is stress, friction, and breakdown. How do I know? I can see it. And so can you.

We'll take a closer look in the next chapter. Seeing the problem is the first step to solving it.

THE BIG 3 SQUEEZE

"The PC creates the illusion that it's doing all the work. It's simply not true. . . . Dozens of muscles, joints, and functions are brought into play and kept in play for hours at a time."

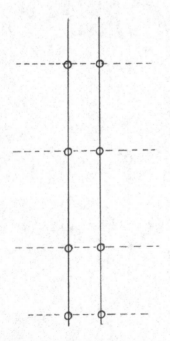

Figure 3.1 The human musculoskeletal grid.

Many people who come to my clinic bring envelopes of Xrays. I try not to look at them. Xrays are deceptive, showing symptoms rather than the source of the problem. The best technology for focusing on the problem comes built into the human skull—your two eyes.

Take a look at figure 3.1. Pretty, isn't she? Or, if you prefer—handsome, isn't he?

I know the illustration looks like a genderless grid, but to me it is the superstructure of a beautiful and functional body. Figures 3.2a and 3.2b will show you what I mean.

Notice how the lines run parallel and form ninety-degree angles exactly at the ankles, knees, hips, and shoulders. Except for the shoulders, those

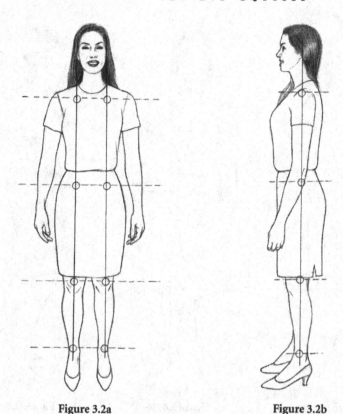

Figure 3.2a   Figure 3.2b

Front and side view of the musculoskeletal superstructure.

angles are also in vertical alignment, and the only reason for the shoulders being an exception is to account for individual size variation.

What we're looking at here is intact, fully functional design range of motion. The woman in the next illustration, figure 3.3, is showing us her individual range of motion. The horizontal lines are no longer parallel, and the ninety-degree angles are not in vertical alignment with the grid. Also, the head seems to have shifted forward and off center. DROM and IROM don't line up.

Figure 3.4 distorts the grid to match the model's musculoskeletal dysfunctions. Figure 3.5 is a side view. See the consequences? The vertical load-bearing capacity of the body achieved by the alignment of the ankle, knee, hip, and shoulders is undermined. In addition the horizontal parallel lines are askew, and with it the balance and stability of the whole structure is radically compromised. Notice the head? It's

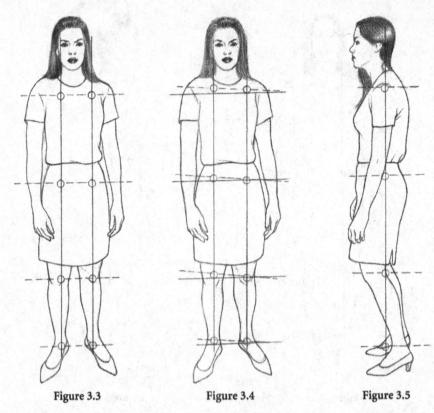

| Figure 3.3 | Figure 3.4 | Figure 3.5 |

The disparity between the solid lines and the grid show the clash between DROM and IROM that leads to dysfunction and chronic joint and muscle pain.

moved forward of the center line. The support system that was directly under it is gone. The weight is jackknifing the spine forward and down.

Now, in figure 3.6, we've eliminated the human form and super-imposed both grids. DROM is solid and IROM is dotted. The disparity between the two is pronounced, and therein lies the problem. If our bones do what the muscles tell them, something is wrong with this illustration. The muscles should be telling the bones to stand erect in vertical and horizontal alignment. But the message is not getting through. The major posture muscles of the model are disengaged to various degrees. To stand, she is using IROM to recruit an array of compensating secondary and primary muscles that are producing a dysfunctional misalignment of the body's superstructure.

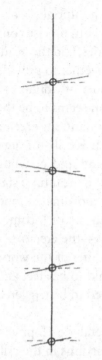

The joints that are involved in this IROM are being subjected to stress, friction, extra impact, and lateral twisting. Some muscles are doing extra work, others hardly any at all. Tendons and ligaments are being yanked on and twisted. And cartilage in the joints receives extra wear and tear.

If you were walking down Fifth Avenue in Manhattan and noticed that Rockefeller Center was tilting at the same angle as our model's body, I guarantee that you'd be out of there in a New York minute. Gone! We'd realize instantly that gravity was about to deposit a load of expensive bricks and mortar in the skating rink. But we look at our own body in the mirror and assume that the basic laws of structural engineering don't apply. Gravity affects a misaligned building, but not the human body?

Dream on! The stresses are even worse because the body moves, a building doesn't.

Figure 3.6
Side view of
joint misalignment.

Imagine a giant hand that reaches down, picks up a minivan as it travels along the highway, squeezes, and then sets it back on the road. The minivan continues on, but everything has changed. The relationship and interactions of the components can't possibly remain the same. The tires wear differently, the shock absorbers have been altered, and the drive train is crimped. The giant hand imposed a new design on the minivan, one that's not likely to do much for reliability or resale value.

IROM does the same thing. But instead of being squeezed by a hand, our bodies are being tranquilized by an ever-motionless environment and then crumpled by gravity.

A Question of Priorities

Roughly speaking, skeletal muscles have three missions: erection, locomotion, and stabilization. I'm not saying that all muscles do all three jobs. Some do, some don't. In general they help us stand upright, walk, run, or make other gross directional movements, and with precise control they move the torso, the lower and upper extremities, and the head. In combination these otherwise-distinct roles work together to provide the necessary finesse to walk, grasp, throw, and—wonder of wonders—operate a computer keyboard and mouse. Locomotion seems to be the precursor to the other two functions. For a newborn infant, the erector and stabilization functions are close to absolute zero. It is only through wiggling and jiggling, flopping and squirming, rolling and crawling that he or she comes to the point of standing up. In the meantime stabilization is jelling as the baby goes from gleefully uncoordinated food disasters to world-class patty-cake. This primitive means of locomotion, sans arms and legs, accesses the posture muscles—the erectors—that will allow her to stand on two feet. (By the way, one of the worst things Mom and Dad can do is hoist the wiggling child to her feet and help her "walk." It's too soon; the posture muscles need to be triggered first.)

What the baby shows us is that musculoskeletal development takes place from the inside out. That's what the contortions in the crib or on the floor are all about. Muscles are arranged in layers, and many of the deepest pairs and groups are responsible for keeping the body erect. Posture muscles maintain their strength and functions like any other muscles—through motion provided by the stimulation of the person's environment. For the baby Mom and Dad are the environment. They tickle, she wiggles. The spinal, hip, and shoulder muscles are stimulated. When she crawls, the same thing happens.

Fully developed structure is lost in the same way. A patient bedridden for a long time can't stand upright, let alone walk. To a lesser extent, the same thing happens to a person stuck at a desk all day. The posture muscles disengage because they aren't being used. With less and less motion being required by the environment, the erectors aren't being stimulated enough to retain their functional capacity. They weaken, and the loss of vertical alignment (I call it "vertical load-bearing") restricts the design range of motion for the load-bearing joints. It's the equivalent of the giant hand squeezing the minivan, but what's being bent is not the axle but our joints.

Because of this restriction and stress, the weakening posture muscles need help. So they recruit other lesser muscles, most of them on the outer periphery of the body, to help keep DROM in a semblance of proper alignment. These recruited muscles are not strong enough or in the right locations to maintain the grid's right angles and parallel lines.

But joint articulation occurs—after a fashion, and at the cost of eventually damaging or destroying the mechanism. In the interest of moving, the body sacrifices proper alignment. Instead of doing one job well, the erector muscles end up doing two jobs poorly: erection *and* locomotion. It's the lesser evil, seeing that if you can't move, you won't be able to hunt or gather food. But lost alignment interferes with movement, which in turn leads to more lost alignment, even less movement, and so on. Eventually, the body can't stand upright and can't move. The lesser evil has become the maximum threat to survival.

> **BALANCING ACT**
>
> Standing upright on two feet isn't easy. It is a major feat of engineering. Balance is everything. To achieve it, the body's major posture joints, or load joints—the ankles, the knees, the hips, and the shoulders—are stacked one atop the other. There are eight of them in pairs of four on each side of the body. Gravity presses down, and there is vertical load-bearing. Furthermore, to balance the load between two feet, the load joints are in horizontal parallel alignment from left to right.

Is that an extreme case? But how many times have you heard about "Poor Joe, he's flat on his back in bed because of a ruptured disk"? Trapped at his desk, Joe's posture muscles—the erectors—gradually lost strength. His skeletal alignment deteriorated, and with it came stress on his joints. He had to keep moving, though, so erector functions were borrowed, and peripheral muscles were brought in to help.

At this point Joe wondered if he was developing carpal tunnel syndrome. His wrist started stiffening. But it wasn't because the keyboard was making an unreasonable demand on his hand and wrist. Those functions would have been fine if they hadn't been also recruited to help keep Joe's shoulders and head from jackknifing forward and smashing into the screen. In other words, individual range of motion was in conflict with design range of motion.

Joe was unaware of the danger at first. He didn't notice the symptoms of disengaged posture muscles. His head and shoulder *gradually* rounded forward. He *gradually* lost the arch in his lower back. Finally, he felt a *gradual* tightening in his wrist that *gradually* started to hurt. Then he bought a wrist brace. (We'll spend more time on braces and other palliatives later in the book, but right now it's enough to know that they are only repositioning the wrist and shifting the stress elsewhere. The pain may go away temporarily, but like Chinese water torture, where the first few drips may go unnoticed, the millionth one causes agony.)

Joe cut back on the number of hours he spent at the keyboard and bought voice-recognition software. He stopped going to the health club and taking walks on the weekends. He could walk all right, but he just didn't feel like it. The worse Joe felt, the less he moved; the less he moved, the worse he felt. Yet at any point, if you asked Joe how he was doing, he'd have shrugged and said, "Fine."

How did Joe end up in the hospital with ruptured disks? He caved in on himself, gradually losing his core muscular strength. Understimulated, Joe's big posture muscles, which are designed to do heavy work, were shut down, and the surface muscles took over. He could move back and forth to the men's room; he could operate his PC. Dutifully, the body contrived to deliver the minimum to keep him moving.

THE OTHER RSI

If you replace the word *repetitive* with *restricted*, it's a more accurate label for these common injuries. By limiting movement to just a few of the same moves that occur over and over again, we are creating musculoskeletal imbalances. The few active muscles strengthen, and the inactive ones weaken. But it would be a mistake to adopt solutions that would attempt to get rid of this restricted movement. The only thing wrong with restricted movement is that it is restricted. It should be augmented with a variety of motion that supports related functions. Ergonomic reengineering and gadgetry fail because the solution amounts to replacing a restricted motion that is causing pain with another restricted motion that isn't causing pain—yet. Eventually it will.

Nevertheless, one day the minimum wasn't enough. Joe's printer was on the floor, and he had to bend over to pick it up and move it. But his weak posture muscles couldn't handle that job. He didn't know that, though. Nor did he suspect that his skeletal misalignment had reached the point that it was severely stressing three of his lumbar disks. Bending over for the printer was the final and *sudden* straw.

He was still wearing the wrist brace when they admitted him to the emergency room.

Joe followed his individual range of motion down a well-worn path that eventually left him "flat on his back." He became *motionally* anorexic. His posture muscles were in need of motion, yet he starved them even more. Like many of us, he probably would argue that he moved constantly. But as a result of his life and work style, Joe was moving only a relatively few muscles (even when he worked out at the gym). For the most part, the muscles that he did move were the smaller, peripheral muscles that could not take the wear and tear. Joe's DROM and IROM fought it out, and he lost.

What we are looking for in this book is motion that promotes and provides design range of motion. It's the only way to restore your musculoskeletal platform, and once that happens, there's no reason you can't swing a hammer or pound a keyboard all day long.

Give and Take

One of the reasons that I deliberately pair hammers and keyboards is that I am still trying to convince you that a PC is a tool. "Yeah, yeah," you're probably thinking, "I work with a PC, so it's a tool." I'm serious. A hammer requires muscle-power. The same goes for a PC's keyboard and mouse. The lack of sweat, blisters, and splinters isn't relevant.

Modern life is very deceptive. We live in such relative luxury that for many of us, "work" seems like it does not require physical effort anymore. Even so-called laborers are using nail guns and power saws. Hold the tool, flip the switch, and let it rip.

Okay. Stop right there. What do you suppose holds the tool? Muscles. But now, instead of fluid hand, wrist, elbow, and shoulder involvement in swinging an old-fashioned hammer, the power tool is being brought to the work and held in position. There's different muscular demand and engagement. Functions that were once involved are being bypassed. A nail gun isn't dainty and light, and carpenters are aware of the physical activity involved (although most of them don't realize that the twinges they feel in their lower back and their neckaches are symptoms of the functions they've lost using a nail gun rather than swinging a hammer). The PC, on the other hand, sits quietly on a stand or desk and creates the illusion that it is doing all the work.

It's simply not true. To operate this high-tech tool, dozens of muscles, joints, and functions are brought into play and kept in play for hours at a time. Typing a single line of the manuscript for this book—about seventy-five keystrokes—took approximately three hundred separate muscular contractions to both flex and extend the fingers of the hand and to abduct and adduct the arms. That's not counting upper-torso movement, arm flexion and extension, and eye muscle activity. Yet we take this muscular demand and engagement for granted. And we should. Our human design range of motion has inspired such confidence that we assume it will always be there when we need it.

However, like Joe's, our individual range of motion isn't up to the job because it has been shaped and determined by the way we live long before we sat down at the keyboard and by what we do away from the keyboard. What DROM giveth, IROM taketh away. It's as if the carpenter went back to swinging a hammer eight hours a day after years of using nothing but the nail gun. The wrist would be flapping, the elbow flying, the shoulder blade sticking out as the body improvised a way to work around inaccessible functions.

The same thing is happening at the PC keyboard. Inside, at the muscular core, there is a vacuum. On the periphery improvisation is running wild. Look around the

---

ABDUCTION/ADDUCTION

Abduction means moving away from a vertical line drawn down the center of the body.

Adduction is the opposite function. The movement is toward the vertical center line.

On a standard keyboard, when the left hand moves left toward the A-key, the arm is abducting. When the right hand moves left toward the space bar, it is adducting.

office at your coworkers. Look in the mirror. Stop the action. Freeze everyone in place. See it?

No? What's your posture like as you read this book?

What should be erect and stable postures are slumping.

Hello, Rockefeller Center.

It's becoming increasingly difficult for people to sit up and stand up straight.

Hello, crumpled minivan.

Old-timers used to say, "That boy will be all right once he fills out." The filling out—from the core to the periphery—isn't taking place. As a result, without the capacity for vertical loading, the body is being pulled forward and down by gravity. All work is movement; as the body slumps toward the horizontal, locomotion becomes harder and harder.

Hello, chronic pain.

THREE CURVES AND YOU WALK

"People with carpal tunnel syndrome have 'blisters' in their wrists . . . caused by the adjustments that are made to skeletal misalignment."

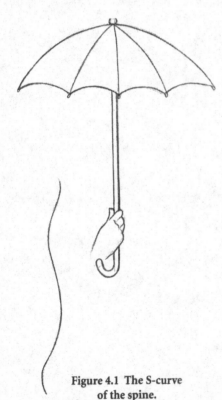

Figure 4.1 The S-curve of the spine.

Uh-oh—the spine, centerfold of serious anatomy texts. Don't worry. All you really need to know about the spine is that when it's healthy and functional, it has the shape of an elongated S. Truly, what you see is how you feel. Take a look at figure 4.1.

The hand and umbrella are props. Focus on that squiggly line to the left—the spinal S-curve. The S seems a little funny at the top, as if somebody stepped on it, but the upper (cervical), middle (thoracic), and lower (lumbar) curves are the important characteristics. They produce a neat balancing act, figure 4.2, that allows the pelvis to hoist the upper torso and head into a vertical position and keep it there.

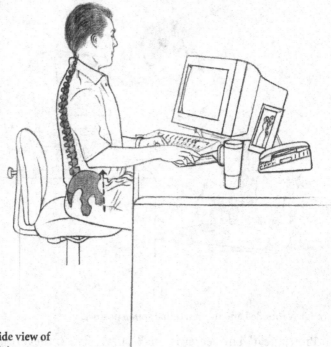

**Figure 4.2 Side view of
spine and pelvis.**

Instead of a stiff tent pole that would need external support to remain
erect, we have a stack of "poker chips"—thirty-three of them—each
separated by a semisoft cushion to act as a shock absorber and to provide flexibility.

There's a hole drilled into the middle of the chips and cushions,
through which the spinal cord travels, branching out here and there to
enervate the muscles and organs.

Poker chips? Cushions? Drilled? Hey, I'm trying to keep it simple.

And it is simple. The spine's form follows its function. The individual vertebrae are intended to work together to bear the weight of the
skull, the shoulder girdle and upper extremities, and the thoracic skeleton (rib cage) containing the organs of the cardiovascular system;
below that the abdominal cavity and the other internal organs hitch a
ride. In short, the spine's job is heavy lifting and heavy balancing. This
load must be kept aloft while the body twists and turns, runs and walks,
stretches, throws, crawls, and dances. At the same time, the spinal column provides a conduit for the main "Information Highway" of the
central nervous system and protects it from damage.

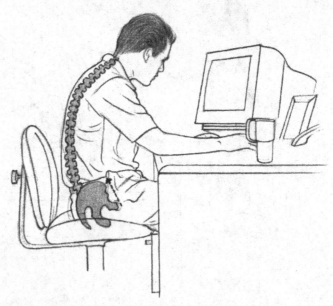

Figure 4.3 A rounded and dysfunctional spinal posture.

Pretty neat! The secret is the S-curve. By cantilevering and counterbalancing those three curves, the structure achieves dynamic flexibility and strength over a wide range of motion. An Alexander Calder mobile uses the same sort of interaction to glide majestically through space. Calder did it with a welding torch. The human body emerged from a different kind of manufacturing process, with individual components that are sized and shaped to form the S-curve. If you found one in pieces under the Christmas tree, it could be re-created easily like a jigsaw puzzle: *Did anybody see a C-7? No, but I have an L-1.*

Match up the right shapes, and the vertebrae all drop neatly into place, but without ligaments, tendons, and muscles, the jigsaw-puzzle spine would be incomplete. The bones of the spine have practically no overall intrinsic strength of their own. Muscles give us *backbone.* In earlier chapters we discussed how dependent muscles are on motion to contract properly and to perform their assigned functions. Spinal muscles are no exception. Most people who are experiencing chronic pain related to a PC are bringing dysfunctional spinal muscles with them to the computer at work, at school, or to kick back and have some fun at home.

The reason is as plain as day. No, make that as plain as the S-curve.

The spine's most vital feature is being replaced by a C. Check out figure 4.3. The three curves have merged into one. As inactive muscle groups throughout the body lose strength and function, they cannot provide direct or indirect support to the spine. The loss of vertical alignment and load-bearing shows up in a rounded back that throws the head and shoulders forward and rolls the butt back and up. Notice how the vertical arrow on the pelvis in figure 4.2 has tipped toward the back as the spine rounds in 4.3.

Move forward to sit on the edge of your chair. Pull your head back, and position your feet and thighs a shoulder-width apart. Try to feel the curve in your lower back. Let your stomach muscles relax. If there is someone else around, ask them to tell you when your head and back are in a vertical line. Now sit there, and time how long it takes for you to become uncomfortable. Instantly? Thirty seconds? Two minutes?

We all should be able to sit in that position indefinitely with no discomfort or fidgeting. When you came out of the position, did your shoulders slump and your hips shift back and down as your lower back lost its curve? If so, you went right back into the C-curve. This is a posture of dysfunction. It's the one you use to drive to work in the morning, sit in the coffee shop for a double espresso, attend meetings, watch a movie, veg out in front of the TV—and operate a PC.

Because it doesn't hurt when we drink the espresso, Starbucks is okay; the coffee won't be blamed. When the pain or stiffness occurs in front of the PC, we know what's what: computer pain syndrome. The difference is that we are working with the PC. Work requires muscle-power, and our muscles are taking the day off—the week, month, year, and the rest of our lives. Eventually, lifting the Starbucks cup will hurt too. Even pleasure requires muscle-power.

A Chain Reaction

Try another experiment. Simply sit in your chair, straighten your back, and then relax it. Do this five or six times. Did you notice that your hips were moving too? If not, place a thumb on each hipbone—the knobs

---

THE CENTRALITY OF NEUTRALITY

In a functional person, going from flexion to extension is like changing the gears in an automobile's manual transmission: The gearshift level passes through neutral before it goes from first gear to second, third, or fourth. Similarly, a muscle takes the joint (any of them, not just the hips) from flexion to neutral, whereupon another muscle takes it from neutral to extension. Neutral, then, is the balance point, where the joint can smoothly open, close, or rotate depending on demand. When the joint is prevented from going into neutral, the body loses balance and vertical alignment because the joint remains locked in either flexion or extension. Try walking without bending your knees. To do it, you're forcing them to stay in extension. The problem is that most people cannot fully relax contracted joint muscles, or, conversely, fully contract relaxed joint muscles. These muscles are either too strong or too weak.

---

on the right and left sides—and then straighten your back and let it slump a couple of times. Your hipbone knobs will make small arcs. Notice that when you relax, your hips slip back and down into the chair. What's happening is that your hips are going into flexion, which they are designed to do. Basically, when sitting or bending at the waist, the top half of the body is allowed to fold toward the bottom half, with the pelvis acting as a big hinge.

Think how useful this capability is. We can tie our shoes, weed our garden, and sit in a chair. In fact, since modern men and women spend so much time sitting down, as opposed to tying shoes and weeding the garden, the hip flexors get a lot of use. These muscles are adept at putting us into that flexed, half-folded position and keeping us there for hours at a time. In the process the spine, riding as it does on the pelvis's sacrum, is pulled into flexion as well.

If you recall, flexors are always paired with extensors. In figure 4.4, the hip flexor and extensor muscles (not shown) are equally matched in strength and function, which puts the hip in a balanced or neutral position, as indicated by the arrow. The spine is also in neutral, as shown by the functional S-curve. But in figure 4.5, since our hip extensor muscles aren't being used nearly as much, the flexors dominate, and the hip and spine begin to spend more and more time in only one place—not in neutral but in flexion. As a result our hip and spinal extensor muscles weaken and disengage. If you compare the two illustrations and note the arrows, you'll see that in figure 4.5 the hip is rolling in a counterclockwise direction toward the rear.

Hence the spine is deprived of its system of countervailing curves, while at the same time being confronted with the problem of holding the head upright without the benefit of vertical alignment. An upright cervical spine (the upper part of the S) acts as a pedestal for the skull. Tip it over by just a few degrees, and a handful of small muscles in the neck, shoulders, and thoracic back (the middle part of the S) are left to carry the unbalanced load.

Imagine trying to balance an elephant on the tip of a fishing pole. Even if the pole were strong enough to support the weight, once it got out of plumb, Jumbo would be heading south, pronto. Luckily, as the head topples, the powerful hip flexors are at one end of the spine holding on—otherwise the C would resemble an inverted U or worse. But the hip flexors have other important work to do, like helping us walk. This conflict produces enormous stress and strain, along with elaborate muscular contortions and compensation in chain reactions all over the body.

Figure 4.4 Hips in neutral position.

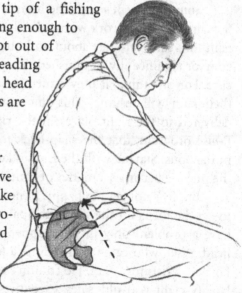

Figure 4.5 Hips in flexion.

HIPS FIRST

Head first. No, hips first. What the brain is to the central nervous system, the pelvic girdle is to the musculoskeletal system. All living creatures have brains (more or less); our pelvis is unique. Without it we wouldn't be able to stand fully erect or even to sit down comfortably. Because of its central location, the pelvis is a major player from head to foot.

Several of the E-cises that I'll be introducing in the next few chapters are designed to help your hips escape from flexion and restore enough extensor function to allow your spine to resume its S-curve. You'll gradually start strengthening and reengaging your underused muscular core.

Many people are perplexed by the idea that therapy focused on the hips can affect hands, wrists, and arms. But the body is a closely integrated unit. A major change in one part of the musculoskeletal system has consequences in every other part of the system. If we can't get the hips out of flexion, the spine's S-curve will never be restored; without the S-curve the head and shoulders remain forward; and that means vertical loading is compromised; and so on, and so on, and so on.

Sound grim? It's not. The body is eager to return to function. In the clinic we often work with individuals who have suffered from joint pain for years, yet after about an hour of E-cise therapy, their pain is gone or significantly diminished. They're amazed. But it's no miracle cure. For one thing, if they return to starving their bodies of motion, their pain will resume. This "motion potion" is so powerful, when delivered to the right places in the right proportions by way of the E-cise program, that the snap-back to good health can seem almost miraculous. Staying with the E-cises keeps the pain at bay. In that way the miracle becomes a matter of routine maintenance.

But let's not get hip happy. I know from experience how hard it is to get the focus off the site of the pain. Most PC users think that they have a problem only in their upper extremities, shoulders, neck, or head. Peter, who came to the clinic a few years ago, was a classic case. His left wrist hurt. Bad. He couldn't use it, which wasn't helpful to a twenty-eight-year-old sales executive in the habit of sending out roughly one hundred e-mails a day to his customers and business team members. You probably know somebody like Peter—or *are* somebody like Peter: a cell phone in one hand, a notebook computer in the other. We put him on an E-cise program, and when the pain abated, he said, "I wonder if that has anything to do with my back?"

"Your back?" I asked. "This is the first you've mentioned it."

"It's hurt for about a year."

"Does it hurt now?"

He gave me a strange look. "No."

Of course the pain was related. The body is a unit. In Peter's case he was rotating his upper torso to the right and lifting his left shoulder in an attempt to ease the friction in his wrist as he typed at the keyboard. With a rounded spine, that maneuver was creating nerve impingement in the lower back.

Sciatica, another common form of nerve impingement, is also hip-related. Long-distance drivers often experience pain in their low back or buttocks because their hips have settled into flexion enough to interfere with the sciatic nerve root that passes through the area. Many people have learned to raise their shoulder or twist laterally in the seat to relieve the pain. As with Peter, the stress is being transferred up the back toward the shoulders, where the stress is not as immediately noticeable. The next time you're at a highway rest stop, take a look at the drivers emerging from cars who are rubbing their shoulders. What they really should be doing is getting their hips out of flexion.

The Wrist Taking of Carpal Tunnel Syndrome

The body is acutely sensitive to friction, and that's why, without thinking about it, we twist and turn, make upper body rotations, cock a shoulder, or perform other adjustments. The basis for this response is perfectly logical: a *temporary* stimulus is provoking *temporary* misalignment of the body. In turn, to minimize stress, the system is making an appropriate *temporary* accommodation. The assumption is that the body will return to alignment and balance. But if that doesn't happen, the temporary arrangements become permanent.

If a blister developed on your right heel, you'd probably start favoring your left leg while walking. There'd be a slight limp caused by prematurely transferring weight into the left hip and flexing and extending the knee more forcefully. That's fine. But if the blister never went away, the friction that you were trying to abate in your right heel would be transferred to your hip and knee joints. Eventually, there would be pain and damage to those joints. In all accuracy, you could say, "I have a blister in my hip and a blister in my knee."

People with carpal tunnel syndrome or other computer-related pain symptoms have "blisters" in their wrists. There is friction and stress. These blisters are not caused by using a PC's keyboard or mouse. They are caused by the adjustments that are made to skeletal misalignment. And they are just as visible as a limp. You can see these adjustments in the position of the head, the shoulders, the wrist, and the hands.

In figure 4.6 the model is seated, which means what? She has lost

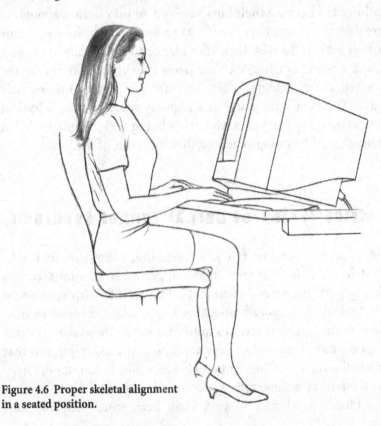

Figure 4.6 Proper skeletal alignment in a seated position.

the use of four of her eight load-bearing joints (knees and ankles). To hold herself in an upright position, she has only her hips and shoulders to work with. In this illustration, no problem—she's fully functional. The head is back and in vertical alignment with the shoulders and hips; her pelvis is strong, and it makes for a stable foundation. But that's not the case in figure 4.7. And there's another difference between the two illustrations. The functional model's head, shoulder, and hip alignment has affected the position of her wrists (figure 4.6). There's an arch; with the palm facing down, the wrist is slightly cambered or arched when placed on a flat surface or held in a horizontal position. Do you see that arch in figure 4.7? It's not there. The elbow has dropped lower as the upper arm's position changed, and the wrist is flat on the desk. Figures 4.8 and 4.9 also show the effect of spine and hip flexion on the wrist position.

Try it yourself. For the moment, ignore the model and sit sideways

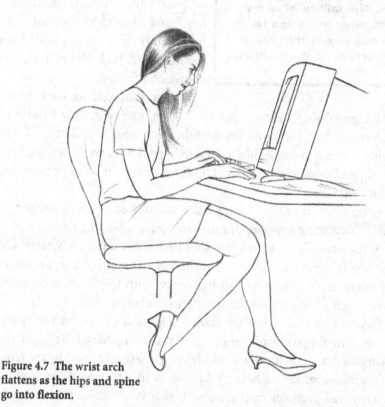

Figure 4.7 The wrist arch flattens as the hips and spine go into flexion.

FIRE

The body is a furnace. It is always burning. That's what metabolism is all about: the breakdown of molecules to produce energy in the form of heat. Therefore the body is sensitive to temperature variations. It has several mechanisms for responding to excess heat generated by friction. One of them is swelling—appropriately known as "inflammation." Swelling is a simple means of restricting the motion that is producing friction. The fallacy of using anti-inflammatory drugs to reduce swelling is that there is no decrease in the friction.

to a table or desk. Place your forearm on the table, running parallel with your thigh, with your palm down and your upper arm and elbow held at a ninety-degree angle. It doesn't matter whether it's your right or left side. Pull your head and shoulders back as far as you can. Feel the S-curve develop its arch in your lower back? Hold that position, and glance down at your wrist without moving your head position. You should see that now there is a space under the wrist immediately behind the palm of your hand. If there isn't, your head and shoulders are not fully back. Make sure to roll your hips forward and tuck them under to counteract flexion.

Got the arch in your wrist? Now, let go. Slump. Allow your back to round and your head and shoulders to come forward. The arch in your wrist will flatten. If you continue to push your shoulder forward and down, you'll feel a growing strain and pressure in the wrist. Pull back on your shoulder, and the pressure will ease.

Although you've been sitting sideways to the table, this position is similar to operating a mouse or other computer pointing device. In figure 4.8, the model's back and shoulder flatten her wrist arch, while the mouse levers the hand upward and increases the tension in the wrist; her spine is in a C-curve. But in figure 4.9, with the S-curve restored, the wrist arch is visible and the wrist tension eases.

Figure 4.10 shows the outline of a hand and the internal bone structure. The fingers or phalanges start at the knuckle of the hand; the metacarpals extend below the knuckles to the wrist, formed by the cluster of eight carpal bones held by ligaments in a transverse arch. It's a relatively small and confined area, isn't it? If you consider the forearm as well as the hand, twenty-nine separate muscles and their tendons share this space. Many of those muscles originate in the forearm, which means that to flex and extend the fingers—each of them has three working joints (the thumb has two)—there isn't much extra room. It's like constant rush-hour traffic getting the tendons threaded through the wrist.

But you know what? In a functional body, there are no fender benders and no gridlock. The tendons and muscles stay in their own lanes. But when skeletal misalignment is present, the traffic in the "carpal tunnel" starts to clog up. That's what you were feeling when I had you roll your shoulder forward until the arch under your wrist flattened.

To experience this in a position more akin to operating a keyboard or mouse, sit forward in a chair with your feet a shoulder-width apart. With your hands palm down on the knees, rest your forearms along the length of the thighs. Ready? Slowly bring your head toward the knees. You'll feel your elbows levering downward on the radius and ulna in the forearm, which are prying upward on the carpal area and squeezing it against the topside of a band of ligaments that encircle the wrist. This is turning your arm bones into levers that are compacting and flattening the carpal area and creating friction on the tendons and nerves that pass through there. Although your thighs are lower than keyboard height, the practical effect is the same in that your hands,

---

HIP ROLLS TO GO

The do-it-yourself examples and E-cises in the book will often ask you to "Roll your hips forward and under." By this I mean for you to take your hips out of flexion and put them into extension. The way to do this is to pull your head and shoulders up and back. You can be either sitting or standing. The upward movement will get your hips to start swinging into position. Now, relax your stomach, and roll your hips forward to create an arch in your back. Don't abruptly snap into this posture, ease into it. Don't worry if it feels stiff or unnatural; that's because your back is used to the flexion-induced C-curve. If there is pain, though, back off the arch until it stops. Hip movement is the key. If your shoulders and head move back without the hips moving forward, you are still in flexion.

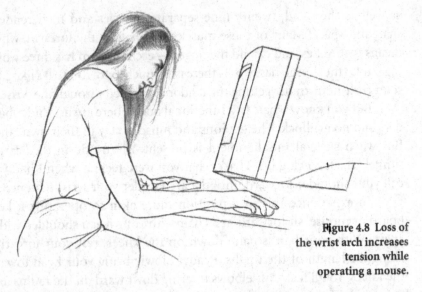

Figure 4.8 Loss of
the wrist arch increases
tension while
operating a mouse.

wrists, and arms will be typing in a parallel position. In both cases the head, shoulders, and back move forward to create a counterweight at the elbows that transmits upward pressure into the wrists.

The mouse isn't involved. Not at all. The pressure is coming from

CTS SYMPTOMS

In most cases it really doesn't matter what you call chronic musculoskeletal pain. After all, we're treating the cause, not the symptoms. For the record, carpal tunnel syndrome symptoms are numbness, tingling, or pain in the area of your thumb, index, middle, and ring fingers. The pain is often worse at night than during the daytime. Other medical conditions can cause these symptoms as well. A wide variety of hand, wrist, and arm symptoms go by different designations. Here again there's a tendency to classify and treat conditions according to where the pain happens to occur. An example is Guyon's canal syndrome. It's a lot like carpal tunnel syndrome, except it's a different nerve passing through a different part of the wrist. But it too is caused by skeletal misalignment, muscular weakness, and structural instability. In my view these various syndromes serve only to demoralize people and convince them that they are suffering from some mysterious disease.

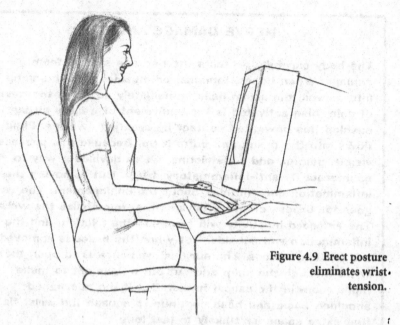

Figure 4.9 Erect posture eliminates wrist tension.

your head, shoulders, and back. And it's constant no matter what you are doing with your wrist and hand: pointing and clicking, typing, jotting a note with a pencil, or holding a coffee cup. As with the limp that compensates for the blister in your heel, the body is making adjustments based on the assumption that the loss of vertical alignment is only temporary. In this case the adjustment is squeezing and flattening the carpal tunnel area. It's no big deal really, if it happens occasionally. The alternative would be to stop the fingers from all movement. Such a drastic measure doesn't seem called for. So the body permits hand movement at the cost of extra friction. That's great, until we ask the muscles of the hand to "limp" for hours at a time—chafing tendons and nerves while thousands of flexions and extensions of the fingers are called for. Soon there is enough friction to set our wrists on fire. And it does.

In the next chapter we'll start on fire fighting and fire prevention.

Figure 4.10 The skeletal structure of the hand.

NERVE DAMAGE AND CTS

The body carefully protects the nervous system from damage. When bones, tendons, or muscles start bumping into nerves, the alarm bells immediately go off in the form of pain. Also activated is the equivalent of a car's airbag to cushion this unwanted contact by creating swelling. Fluid flows into the tissue and puffs it up. Because this process is visible, painful, and constricting, we've devised a way to counteract it—anti-inflammatory drugs. But removing the inflammation does nothing about the impingement. The same goes for braces or other devices that immobilize the wrist. The enforced inactivity will eliminate the friction, and the inflammation will subside. But when the brace is removed, the friction returns. The surgical response is to open the wrist through the palm and cut out a ligament to make more room in the carpal tunnel. But if the misaligned shoulder, back, and head continue to squash the wrist flat, that extra space isn't likely to last long.

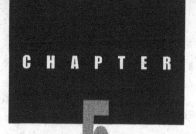

FIVE E-CISE PIECES

"Every minute spent using a computer is a minute of extremely restricted movement."

Effective health care is eight parts diplomacy and two parts therapy. An important aspect of the diplomacy is persuading you to take action. If I can't do that, I've failed—and I hate to fail.

This book presents five therapy programs that I've specifically developed for people who use PCs. The backbone of each of them—to choose an appropriate metaphor—is formed by a series of exercises that target specific musculoskeletal dysfunctions or clusters of dysfunctions. These E-cises, as we call them in the clinic, are simple and easy to do on your own. They don't require special equipment beyond a few rolled-up towels, a pillow, a chair, and the like.

To determine which program is best for you, simply calculate the number of hours you spend using a PC. One to three hours a week is my standard for occasional PC users, one hour a day for moderate users, and from one to two hours a day or more—much more—for power PC users.

By dividing the therapeutic process into categories based on how much time you spend working or playing with a PC, I'm bowing to reality. I know all too well that treatment usually starts where and when pain begins. At the same time, there is usually a misleading cause-and-effect motivator: "I'm on my PC ten hours a day, and boy does my wrist hurt!"

Rather than fight this flawed logic, I've decided to go with the flow and link therapy to PC usage. It will allow you to conveniently slot yourself into a relevant category. Does that mean the PC is causing the pain?

I've said it several times already, and to put it diplomatically again—no!

You can use the PC for five minutes a day and still be in agony. Fortunately for Silicon Valley, you probably won't make a cause-and-effect connection to one of their products. The blame will fall—incorrectly—on something else. The toll-taker at the Delaware Memorial Bridge blames his backache on reaching out to the passing cars; the horticulturist at the Arnold Arboretum in Boston says the rose clippers hurt her wrist; the checker at Vons in Del Mar complains that the cash register is wrecking his thumbs. As a diplomat and a therapist, I suggest we just forget about cause and effect and work on a solution instead.

So if you're in musculoskeletal pain right now, or have episodes of pain, you should turn to chapter 6, where there's a program for pain sufferers in every category, no matter how much or how little you use a PC.

If you are not in pain, you'll need to turn to the chapter that corresponds to the amount of time you use the PC. These E-cise programs are purely prevention.

If you are an occasional user, turn to chapter 7; a moderate user, turn to chapter 8. If you fall into either of these categories, you do not rely on the PC as a primary means of livelihood. The occasional user is dabbling in cyberspace, learning the ropes, and perhaps being taught the ropes by their power-user children. The moderate user, however, is in deeper. Those who spend an hour a day on the computer are probably employing it as both a tool and a toy: sending and receiving e-mail, checking company inventory records, or playing a game to unwind in the evening.

Power users should turn to chapter 9. They need the PC to make a living or, if they are students, to make the grades to make a living. They also use the computer for recreation as well as work. And some kids have become power users because they are addicted to the games, chat rooms, and the Internet "mall."

Time is of the essence. Every minute spent using a computer is a minute of extremely restricted movement. This fact alone is what determines which E-cises are deployed for the various categories. Someone who spends hours in front of a computer cannot expend those hours pursuing a wider, more varied range of motion. Higher-impact E-cises with a greater stimulation value are necessary, as a result. On the other hand, occasional and moderate users do not require as forceful an intervention because they are getting stimulation for their muscles and functions from non-PC sources. The whole purpose for all three of these categories is pain prevention.

And if you're in pain, the E-cise program in chapter 6 combines restoration and recuperation. In that case time is not the key factor. If the supply of motion provided by one's environment is in short supply for whatever reason, an hour a week on the computer or less could be enough to trigger pain.

One final program is offered in chapter 11 to supplement your regular fitness routine and favorite forms of recreation.

E-cise Preview

I've always believed that readers have the right to read a book any way they want—start at the end, graze spontaneously, or whatever. But as an author, I'd like to suggest that you read through the rest of the book before embarking on an E-cise program. I think you'll come away with a clearer picture of both the problem and the solution.

Whatever you decide, let me quickly run through some important points about doing the E-cises:

- The program will not work if you don't do it. Set aside time each day for the E-cises. Their effect is cumulative.

- Do the entire program from beginning to end in the order presented. The sequence builds on itself.

- Don't pick and choose among the E-cises for those that seem to address your concerns. If you are worried about your wrist or elbow, remember that the site of the pain (or stiffness) is usually not the source.

- Do the E-cises every day. An occasional day off is acceptable, but longer breaks mean that you are losing ground.

- Relax your stomach muscles while doing the E-cises.

- Remember to breathe, and breathe from your diaphragm.

After I present the four main E-cise programs in chapters 6 through 9, I then discuss eyestrain and nonpain symptoms like dehydration and obesity in chapter 10; show you how to break out of the workplace jail in chapter 11; answer frequently asked questions in chapter 12; and expose the folly of surgery, painkilling drugs, and ergonomic reengineering in chapter 13.

CHAPTER 6

E-CISES FOR THOSE IN PAIN

```
┌─────────────────────────────────────┐
│          HOME THERAPY               │
│                                     │
│   • Gravity Drop                    │
│   • Sitting Knee Pillow Squeezes    │
│   • Static Wall                     │
│   • Sitting Floor                   │
│   • Pelvic Tilts                    │
│   • Hip Crossover                   │
│   • Pelvic Tilts                    │
│   • Three-Position Toe Raises       │
│   • Sitting Cats and Dogs           │
└─────────────────────────────────────┘
```

I'd love it if this turned out to be the least-read chapter in the book. But I'm not about to make a bet on it. According to the National Institute of Occupational Safety and Health, 20 percent of those who work with computers have some degree of repetitive stress injury. These figures are bound to go higher as the total pool of computer users grows, and as the general population itself becomes less and less functional due to our motion-starved environment.

Ironically, if PCs were banned from the home and workplace tomorrow, this alarming chronic pain trend would continue to rise anyway. We'd just have to assign another coincidental subset: *30 percent of all VCR remote-control users suffer from some degree of repetitive stress injury.* Name the technological device or tool, and if it requires movement from a dysfunctional user, it can and will be blamed for causing injury.

To me, that's the most alarming pain trend of all.

If you are experiencing pain, drop the E-cise menu that matches your PC user profile and perform the one below. You'll find it helpful to review the instructions in chapter 5, and if you jumped here without reading chapters 1 through 4, I suggest you go through that material before beginning the E-cises.

I know. It hurts, and the sooner it stops hurting, the better. But plunging directly into the E-cise program will cheat you in two ways. First, you won't have the necessary background to understand what the body is telling you with pain and how the Egoscue Method helps you to deal with it. Second, when the pain goes away, you'll be more inclined to immediately stop doing the E-cises—*no pain, no problem.* But that's wrong. The problem has been building over the long term, and it requires a long-term solution.

How long? It's hard to be precise because of variations in the extent and interrelationships of individual musculoskeletal dysfunctions. In the clinic it's very rare for a client to leave after an hour or two of his or her first E-cise–based therapy program without showing major improvement. The pain may linger, but it steadily decreases as the program continues. You should experience a similar de-escalation of pain over several days.

When the pain abates for two full weeks, you can begin to switch over to the power PC user's home therapy menu. Although you may use a computer only occasionally, the pain indicates that your work and lifestyle are not providing enough motion to maintain proper musculoskeletal function. The power PC user's E-cise program will help counteract this motion deficit. I want you to ease into the transition by using the power PC user menu one day a week on week three (that's one week after two full weeks of being without pain), two days on week four, three days on week five, four days on week six, and five days on week seven. At that point the ratio will be five days of the power PC user menu and two days of the pain menu. This will be your permanent program. If the pain returns, resume a full seven-day program with the pain menu until you again establish a two-week pain-free window.

If there are setbacks, it helps to ask these questions:

- Have I been doing my E-cise program every day?

- Have I been doing the full program?

- Have I been following the instructions carefully?

- Have I changed the amount or type of physical activity that's occurring?

Many people intend to faithfully do their E-cises, but other commitments get in the way. You have to treat your health—particularly when there's pain—as your number one priority.

I strongly urge you not to succumb to the temptation to pick out a few E-cises and customize your own program. It's important to do the entire menu in sequence. Dysfunctions come in layers and in clusters. The sequence is designed to systematically restore functions that serve as gateways to deeper or more inaccessible layers or clusters of dysfunction.

If an E-cise is difficult to do, stay with it. The difficulty is a measure of the magnitude of the dysfunction that it is attacking. It will get easier as you go along. But if the E-cise causes an increase in pain, stop and temporarily drop it from the routine. Try it again in a day or two; you may find that there's no longer a problem. The other E-cises may be sufficient to change the musculoskeletal interactions to allow the other to be brought back into play.

If there is *no* improvement, consider this important question: If a method that's been so successful treating musculoskeletal disorders is ineffective—and if pain is a symptom—are you actually suffering a musculoskeletal problem, or is it something else? The continuing pain may be the symptom of another condition.

As for my point about making sure you follow the instructions, it probably doesn't need much further explanation. But it is often helpful to have someone else watch you perform the E-cises and compare what you're doing with the instructions that appear in the book.

Finally, pain can return when there is a sudden increase in the amount of physical activity or a change in the type of activity. The E-cises will make you feel better, and when that happens, it is only natural to want to start doing more. "No pain! I can dust off the PC and pull a bunch of all-nighters and weekenders" is the typical reaction. But resist it. Go easy. Gradually, build up the demands you are putting on your body so that your muscles have a chance to strengthen.

Unlike the other E-cise programs, I'm offering one menu for home use only. Why? If you are in pain, the place to be is home. No business as usual, please. I said it earlier—your health is the number one priority. When the pain abates and you've made a transition to the program for power PC users, it is then appropriate to use its office therapy menu.

E-CISE TIPS

- Follow the menu in sequence.
- Don't pick and choose among E-cises. Do all of them in order.
- Honor the body's bilateral design by repeating the E-cises equally on both sides.
- Stop if the E-cise causes pain.
- Keep a slow, steady pace.
- Do at least one of the menus, home or office, once a day. Doing both would be ideal.
- If you miss a day or two, don't worry. Miss three or more—worry!
- On any given day, once you've run through the entire office therapy menu, feel free to take spontaneous E-cise breaks by choosing whichever one seems appropriate to the work you've been doing or the way your body is feeling.

Home Therapy
Total Time: 15 minutes
Frequency: Daily
Special Note: Drop E-cise(s) if pain increases

• GRAVITY DROP

This E-cise (figure 6.1) promotes hip stability and releases the muscles of the thoracic back.

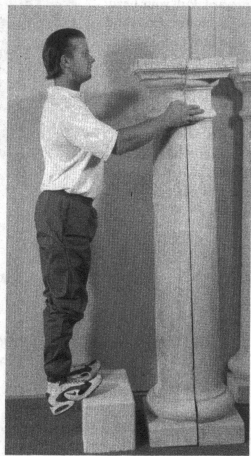

Figure 6.1

Wearing rubber-soled shoes for traction, stand on a step or stairway as though you were climbing upward. Your feet are parallel on the same step and a shoulder-width apart. Arch your back. With one hand, hold on to the railing or another solid object for support, and edge backward until your heels are off the step and hanging in midair. Keep easing back so that more than half of each foot is off the step. Make sure your feet remain parallel, pointing straight ahead, and that they are a shoulder-width apart. Let the weight of your body press down into your heels to engage the posterior muscles of the leg. Don't bend your knees. Keep your head and shoulders back. Hold for three minutes.

● SITTING KNEE PILLOW
  SQUEEZES

This E-cise (figure 6.2)
strengthens and stabilizes
the pelvis.

  Sit on the edge of a
chair, and arch your back
by rolling your hips
forward. Pull your head
and shoulders back, and
make sure your knees and
feet are in alignment with
your hips. Place a foam
block, thick pillow, or
folded seat cushion
between your knees; you'll
need something six to eight
inches thick. Using your
inner thighs, squeeze the

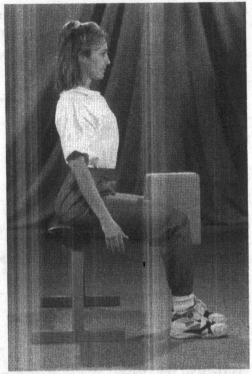

Figure 6.2

Figure 6.3

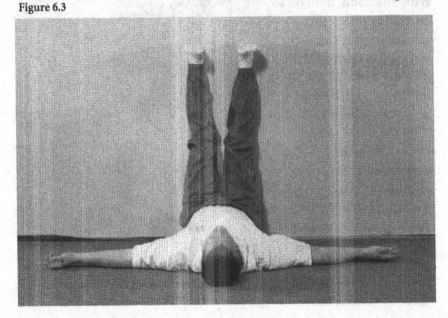

pillow, hold for a half beat, and release it gently. Do a total of forty squeezes, in four sets of ten. Your feet stay parallel and a hip-width apart. Don't let your stomach, upper back, or shoulders participate.

• STATIC WALL

This E-cise (figure 6.3) releases the muscles of the torso, repositions the shoulders, and promotes hip stability.

Lie on your back at the foot of a wall. Place your legs straight up against the wall (so that your upper torso and legs are at ninety degrees), with your feet a hip-width apart. Tighten your thighs, and flex your toes and feet back toward the floor. Get your buttocks and hamstrings (the posterior of the thighs) as close to the wall as you can. The smaller the gap, the better. But if your hips come off the floor, back off until they are flat. Concentrate on relaxing your upper body. Keep the toes flexed equally on each foot, and don't let the feet flare out of parallel. Hold this position for three to five minutes.

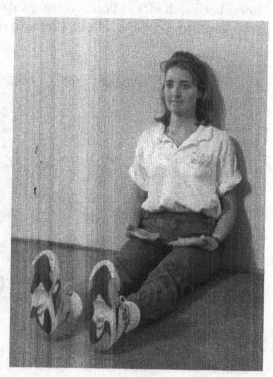

• SITTING FLOOR

This E-cise (figure 6.4) establishes proper engagement of the muscles of the trunk, causes shoulder retraction to strengthen the upper body, and stabilizes the hips.

Sit on the floor with

Figure 6.4

your back against a wall and your legs straight out in front of you. Your feet should be a hip-width apart. Squeeze your shoulder blades together, and hold. Do not lift or cock your shoulders. Keep your head back, tighten your thighs, and flex your feet so your toes are pointing back toward you. Your arms can be at your sides or relaxed atop your thighs. Hold this position for four to six minutes.

• PELVIC TILTS

This E-cise (figures 6.5a and b) strengthens and releases the muscles of the torso.

Lie on your back with your knees bent, your feet flat on the floor, and your hands resting at your sides, palms up. Roll your hips toward your head to flatten your lower back into the floor (a). Do not lift your hips off the floor. Then roll your hips away to make the lower back arch off the floor, creating a space between the floor and your back (b). Do these rolls in a smooth continuous motion as you

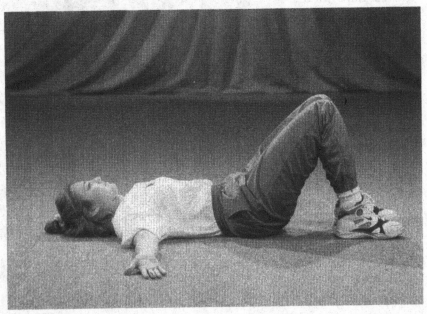

Figure 6.5a

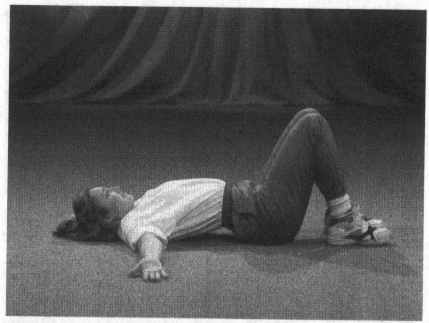

Figure 6.5b

flatten and arch the back. Remember to breathe in sync with the hip movement—inhale up, exhale down. Do ten tilts. Don't move your feet or flap your knees.

• Hip Crossover

This E-cise (figures 6.6a and b) encourages external rotation of the femur (the thigh bone), thereby strengthening and stabilizing the pelvis.

    Lie on your back with both knees bent and your feet flat on the floor. Cross your left ankle over your right knee, and press the left knee out toward the feet (a). While maintaining this position, lower your left foot to the right side and place it flat on the floor (b). The right knee stays bent, and both feet are on the floor. Keep the left knee pressing up toward the ceiling to feel a stretch in the area of your left hip. Hold this position for thirty seconds to one minute. Come out of this the same way you went in. Then reverse the directions and repeat on the other side.

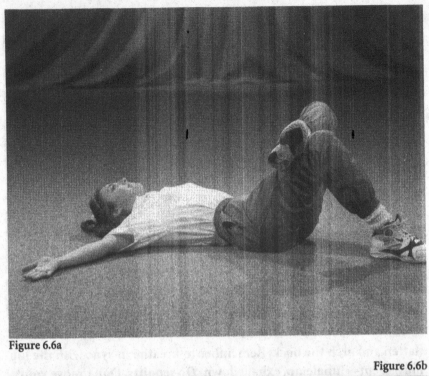

Figure 6.6a

Figure 6.6b

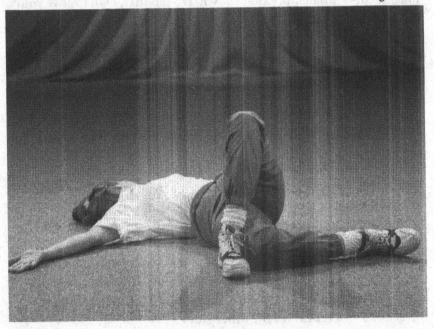

• Pelvic Tilts

Let's do a second set for good measure, now that we've worked on the rotation of the femur. This E-cise demands that the muscles of your torso relax and contract, relax and contract, instead of staying locked in contraction.

Use the E-cise instructions and photos on pages 54 and 55 (figures 6.5a and b).

• Three-Position Toe Raises

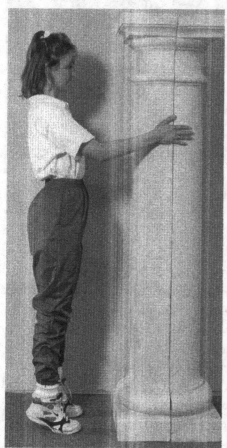

Figure 6.7a

This E-cise (figures 6.7a, b, and c) runs both hips through the full flexion-neutral-extension cycle.

Position one (a): Near a closed door or wall, stand with your feet a hip-width apart and parallel. Pull your head and shoulders back, and roll the hips forward into extension to arch the lower back. Raise up on your toes, keeping your weight evenly distributed on both feet and your knees straight. Come straight up, don't rock forward. Make sure your weight isn't sloshing to the inside or outside of the feet; keep it even. Raise and lower yourself ten times.

Position two (b): Pull your head and shoulders back, and roll your hips forward into extension to arch the lower back. This time your feet

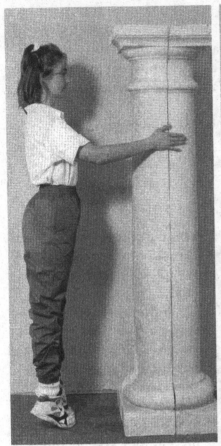

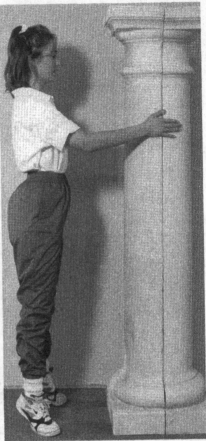

Figure 6.7b

Figure 6.7c

should be pigeon-toed, with the big toes touching. Set the heels a hip-width apart, and angle your toes inward until they touch. Check the stance to make sure your weight is balanced between the two feet and distributed evenly over both feet. Keep the arch in your back. Raise and lower yourself ten times.

Position three (c): Stand in extension with your heels together and your feet spread like a duck with the toes pointed out. Raise and lower yourself ten times. Do these slowly to prevent your feet from rolling to the inner or outer edges.

• SITTING CATS AND DOGS

This E-cise (figures 6.8a and b) builds on the last by reuniting the hips to the spine and shoulders during flexion and extension.

Sit in a chair with your feet flat on the floor, parallel, and about a hip-width apart. Don't lean back, but sit forward toward the front. Rest your hands palms-down by your thighs. Slowly pull your head, shoulders, and hips back into extension. Feel the arch in your lower back as your head moves back to the rear. Head, hips, and shoulders should be aligned and pointing straight at the ceiling (a). When you get there, pause for half a beat, and slowly relax, letting the back round forward and the shoulders, neck, and head come with it (b). We want the back to leave extension—but don't actually force your upper torso farther than its natural stopping point, where the muscles are fully relaxed. Link each Cat and Dog into a smooth, continuous series. Your hands will track back and forth on top of your thighs. Do ten. Remember to breathe.

Figure 6.8a

Figure 6.8b

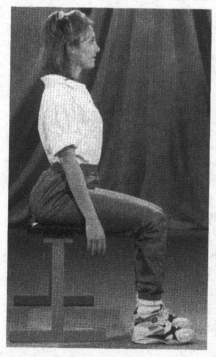
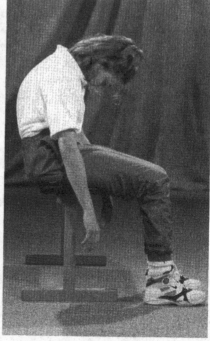

E-CISE MENU FOR OCCASIONAL COMPUTER USERS

HOME THERAPY	OFFICE THERAPY
• Arm Circles	• Standing Chair Stretch
• Elbow Curls	• Sitting Overhead Extension
• Foot Circles and Point Flexes	• Standing Quad Stretch
• Sitting Floor Twist	• Sitting Cats and Dogs
• Cats and Dogs	• Sitting in Extension
• Kneeling Groin Stretch	
• Upper Spinal Floor Twist	
• Cats and Dogs	
• Downward Dog	
• Air Bench	

What I'm offering here is designed as a way for people who use computers for up to roughly three hours a week to avoid problems. Although this usage amounts to only about twenty-five minutes a day, it's time enough to check e-mail, look at the weather report, and do a little on-line shopping. Clearly, the PC is being used not as a major tool, but just enough to make a difference to your musculoskeletal system. Twenty-five minutes of extra demand a day are being put on a system that is already in need of structural stability, muscular strength, and skeletal alignment.

E-CISE TIPS

- Follow the menu in sequence.
- Don't pick and choose among E-cises. Do all of them in order.
- Honor the body's bilateral design by repeating the E-cises equally on both sides.
- Stop if the E-cise causes pain.
- Keep a slow, steady pace.
- Do at least one of the menus, home or office, once a day. Doing both would be ideal.
- If you miss a day or two, don't worry. Miss three or more—worry!
- On any given day, once you've run through the entire office therapy menu, feel free to take spontaneous E-cise breaks by choosing whichever one seems appropriate to the work you've been doing or the way your body is feeling.

Home Therapy
Total Time: 20 minutes
Frequency: Daily

• ARM CIRCLES

This E-cise (figures 7.1a and b) is a ball-and-socket booster. Shoulder joints are bifunctional—they hinge forward and back, and they rotate in a ball-and-socket configuration. Using a mouse or keyboard means a lot of hinge demand, which often locks the shoulder in the forward position. This can happen in either the right or left shoulder—or both at the same time. Arm Circles counteract that tendency.

Stand with your head up, feet parallel about a hip-width apart, and arms at your sides. Curl the fingers of each hand into a light fist with your thumbs straight. (This is known as a "golfer's grip.") Raise your arms out to your sides, keeping the elbows and arms straight, palms down, and your thumbs pointing forward (a). Lift your arms until they are level with your shoulders. If one shoulder

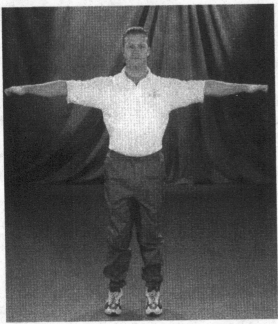

Figure 7.1a

wants to pop up or swing forward, lower both until they stay level. (Pay attention to this, too, when you start doing the circles). Now squeeze your shoulder blades together slightly, and rotate the arms forward in the direction the thumbs are pointing. Make a roughly six-inch-diameter circle. Keep your wrists and elbows straight—the circles must come from the shoulders. Do this twenty-five times at a slow to moderate pace.

Reverse the circles by turning the palms up and thumbs back (b). Crank the thumbs around so that your palms are level. Do another twenty-five. Then repeat back the other way for another twenty-five, and repeat again with the same count to the rear, so that you do a total of fifty in each direction. Remember to breathe.

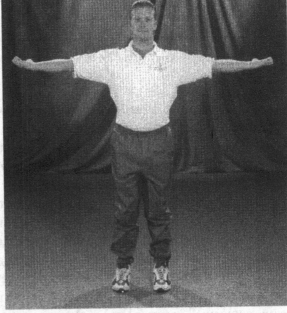

Figure 7.1b

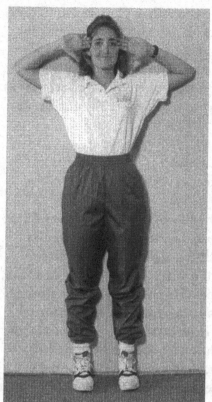

Figure 7.2a

• ELBOW CURLS

This E-cise (figures 7.2a and b) "oils" the shoulder's hinge function. It also protracts and retracts the shoulder blades across the rib cage, to prevent them from getting too comfortable in the forward position as you lean toward the PC. They are harder than they look. Take your time. The photo shows the model against a wall, but with this E-cise I want you to move away from the wall.

Figure 7.2b

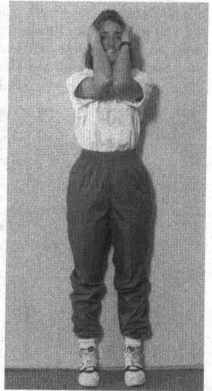

Stand with your feet parallel, a hip-width apart. With your hands in the golfer's grip (see Arm Circles), place the flat area on the back of the index and middle fingers, between the first and second knuckle joints, on the temples in front of your ears; the thumbs extend downward, parallel with the cheeks. Draw your elbows back evenly and in line with the shoulders (a). Don't allow one shoulder to be lazy and not come all the way back. From this starting position, slowly swing your elbows forward until they touch in front (b). Keep your knuckles touching your temples, the thumbs fully extended. Your head should stay erect, not wobble or seesaw. Equalize the work and tension in both sides. Breathe deeply. Do twenty-five Elbow Curls. Each time your elbows touch counts as one curl. If you can't do twenty-five at first, reduce the number and slowly build up to it.

• FOOT CIRCLES AND POINT FLEXES

Now that we've worked on your shoulders, this E-cise (figure 7.3) prepares your ankles to join the load-bearing team. It promotes blood flow, which is impeded by sitting at your PC. Muscular contraction and relaxation assist the heart with its pumping action, particularly in the lower extremities. This E-cise also strengthens the pelvis to better support the body in a fully upright posture.

Lie on your back with one leg extended flat on the floor and the other bent toward your chest with your foot off the floor. Clasp your hands behind your bent knee for support, and circle the foot clockwise thirty times. Meanwhile, keep your other foot on the floor

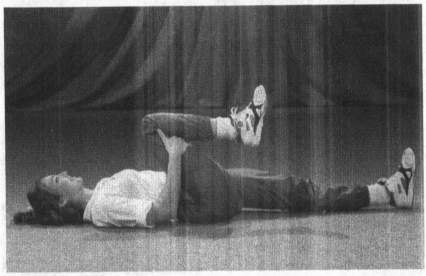

Figure 7.3

with the toes pointed straight toward the ceiling. It's not necessary to flex this foot, just keep it straight. When you've done thirty circles, reverse the direction of the circling foot and repeat for another thirty. Change legs, and circle the other foot clockwise thirty times, then counterclockwise thirty times. Make sure the knees stay absolutely still, with the movement coming from the ankle, not the knee. The pace should be slow to moderate. Do the Foot Circles on both legs, in both directions, before starting the Point Flexes.

For Point Flexes, after completing the last set of circles, stay in the same position on your back with one leg extended and the other bent at the knee and held off the ground with your hands clasped behind your knee. On this leg—the one that is bent—bring your toes back toward the shin to flex. Then reverse the direction to point your foot. Do it twenty times. Switch legs, and repeat another twenty times.

• SITTING FLOOR TWIST

Figure 7.4

Because the PC is directly in front of you, you tend to stay in flexion while work is under way, which puts the spine and hip-extensor muscles under stress. This E-cise (figure 7.4) counters the propensity for the extensors to lose bilateral strength and function. As you can see, the twisting action wrings out both sides equally.

Sit on the floor with

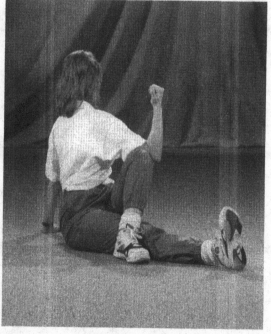

your legs extended in front. Bend your left leg, and cross it over the right knee. Keep the left foot flat on the floor and running parallel to the right leg. The right foot should be pointed at the ceiling. Place your right elbow outside your left knee, twisting the torso to the left. Your head is now facing the rear. Tighten the thigh muscles of the straight leg, and flex the ankle-foot of this leg toward the knee. Place your left hand behind you on the floor for support. Put an arch in your lower back. Hold for one minute (with the ankle-foot flexed), then repeat on the other side. Remember to breathe. Exhaling and inhaling smoothly helps the flexor muscles to relax and allows the extensors to contract.

● CATS AND DOGS

This E-cise (figures 7.5a and b) provides total range of motion in the pelvis and the back in an anatomically correct and safe manner.

Figure 7.5a

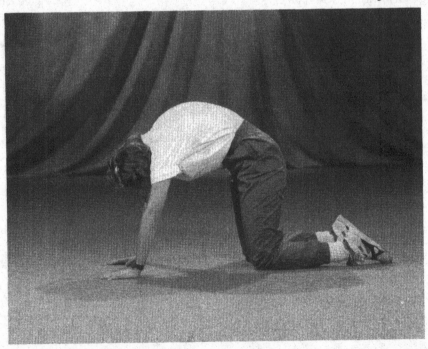

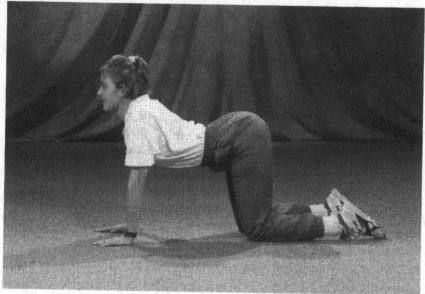

Figure 7.5b

It promotes breathing and better circulation. It's very effective, as you may know if you've done yoga.

Get down on the floor on your hands and knees. Make a "table" by aligning your hands under your shoulders and your knees and thighs under your hips. Your arms should be straight and your thighs parallel to them. Keep your legs and feet parallel to each other, as well. The feet are relaxed and resting across the top side of the toes, not flexed or up on the toes. Make sure your weight is distributed evenly. Smoothly round your back upward as your head curls under, to create a curve that runs from the buttocks to the neck—this is a cat with an arched back (a). Smoothly sway the back down while bringing your head up—this is the perky dog (b). Make these two moves continuously back and forth—don't keep them choppy and distinct. Do one set of ten. Exhale as you move into the cat position, inhale during the dog. Make sure, with the dog, that your head comes fully back and up so that you are looking straight ahead and your shoulder blades collapse toward each other. Take your time. The pace should be slow, but not so slow that it breaks the flow between the cat and dog positions.

• KNEELING GROIN STRETCH

You should feel this E-cise (figure 7.6) in the groin area, thighs, and hips. It releases tension and builds strength.

Kneel on the floor. Extend your left leg with the left foot flat on the floor and placed about two to three feet in front of your body. Get your foot out far enough so that your bent knee is behind your left ankle. Keep both knees and feet a hip's-width apart, without twisting your torso to the left or right. With your head up and back straight, put your interlaced hands palm-down on top of your left knee, and lunge forward. The hands are there for balance and to keep your shoulders square. The lunge will carry your left knee forward to a point directly over your left ankle. We don't want the knee to go beyond the ankle. If it does, your left foot needs to be moved farther out in front of your body. Feel the stretch in the hips, groin, and thigh. Hold this position for one minute. Repeat on the other side.

Figure 7.6

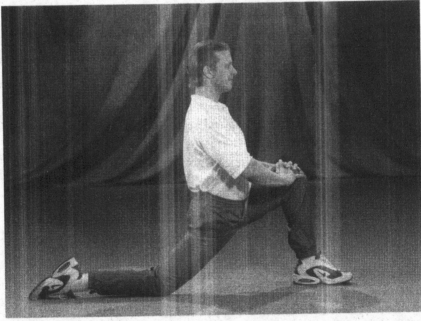

• UPPER SPINAL FLOOR TWIST

This E-cise (figure 7.7) puts the neck, arms, and shoulders on the same plane, where they belong in order to interact properly.

Lie on your side with your knees together and bent. This will put your knees at a right angle to your trunk. Keeping the elbows straight and the palms together, extend both arms along the floor, level with your shoulders, in the direction of your knees, parallel with the bent legs. Slowly lift the upper arm up and over to rest behind you on the floor palm-up, while you turn your head to face the ceiling. Adjust this arm position, if necessary, by finding a shoulder slot that's comfortable. Relax and breathe deeply. Allow gravity to settle the extended arm to the floor along its entire length, from fingers to shoulder. Meanwhile, make sure the knees don't slide apart. You can hold them in place with the other hand (as the model is doing). When the shoulders have leveled out (it may take several minutes and perhaps several sessions to achieve this fully), lift the extended arm and return it to the starting position while exhaling. Hold for at least three minutes, or longer if you have the time and the shoulder hasn't come down onto the floor. Repeat on the other side.

Figure 7.7

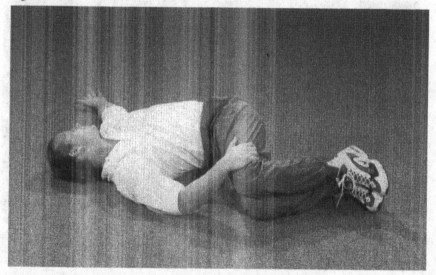

• CATS AND DOGS

Yes, we're going to do this one again.

See E-cise instructions and photos on pages 66–67 (figures 7.5a and b).

• DOWNWARD DOG

Downward Dog (figures 7.8a and b) uses all the extensor functions on the backside of your body. It's also great for colon and bladder functions, which are compromised by prolonged sitting.

Assume the dog position (see Cats and Dogs) (a). Now curl your toes under, and push with your legs to raise your hips and torso, until you are off your knees and your weight is being supported by your hands and feet. Keep pushing until your hips are higher than your shoulders and have formed a tight stable triangle. Your knees should be straight, your calves and thighs tight (b). Don't let your feet flare outward; keep them pointing straight ahead in line with the hands, which need to stay in place—no creeping! Your back

Figure 7.8a

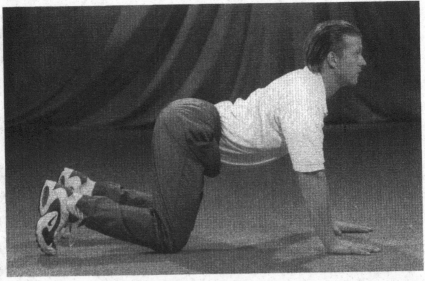

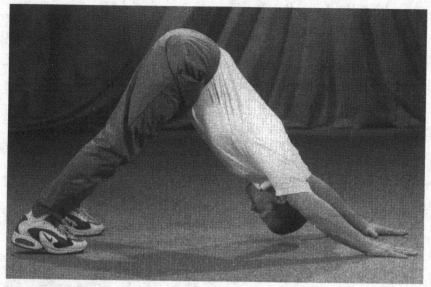

Figure 7.8b

should be flat, not bowed, as the hips push up to create the triangle. Breathe. If you cannot bring your heels flat onto the floor, don't force them. Contract the muscles slowly and steadily to their natural stopping point. You'll know it when you get there. Hold for one minute. It may take several days or weeks to get the heels flat. The muscles will contract a little more each time.

• AIR BENCH

The Air Bench (figure 7.9) promotes lower-leg, thigh, and hip strength, and it relaxes the muscles of the torso. These are all functions we need to be pain free at the PC.

The best way to get into the starting position is to stand with your back to a wall. Press your hips and the small of your back into the wall. At the same time, walk your feet forward and simultaneously slip down the wall surface into a sitting position. Stop when you've reached approximately a ninety-degree angle. Your knees should be over your ankles, not your toes. (You should be able to see your toes.) If you feel pain in your kneecaps, raise your body up the wall to relieve the pressure. Press the low back and midback against the wall, and feel the quadriceps working along the tops of the thighs. Hold for three minutes. Breathe. This can be a struggle. You can start by doing the Air Bench for a few seconds and build to a minute, extend it to two, and then go for three. I've worked with NFL running backs who couldn't get beyond ten seconds at first. When you are finished, scoot back up the wall and walk around for a few minutes.

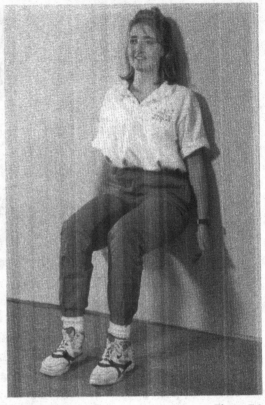

Figure 7.9

Office Therapy
Total Time: 5 minutes
Frequency: At least twice a week
Special Note: Remove your shoes

• STANDING CHAIR STRETCH

This E-cise (figure 7.10) relaxes the muscles of the thoracic back by encouraging hip and lumbar extension, then tops that off with a proper shoulder position. The limited range of motion needed to operate a PC—and most other modern devices—isn't enough to stimulate this interaction.

Place one foot on the seat of a chair with your knee bent and the other foot on the floor. (This leg is straight.) Both feet should be pointed straight ahead. Lean your hips and torso toward the chair so that your front knee is over your ankle. Interlace your fingers, place your hands on the back of your head, and push your elbows back. Do not shrug your shoulders. Make sure your back leg remains straight throughout the exercise. Breathe. Hold this position for thirty seconds. Repeat on the other side.

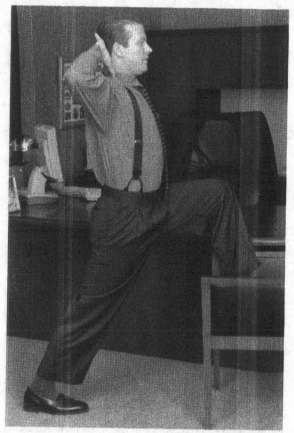

Figure 7.10

• SITTING OVERHEAD EXTENSION

By reaching out toward a keyboard or mouse and holding that position, the scapula (part of the shoulder blade) protracts and stays that way. It needs encouragement to retract. A pilot doesn't fly his plane with the wheels down. You shouldn't fly your PC with your shoulder blades hanging out. This E-cise (figure 7.11) delivers hip extension, relaxes the anterior muscles of the torso, and promotes scapular retraction in the shoulder.

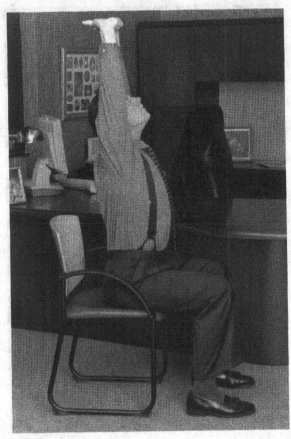

Sit in a chair with your feet flat on the floor, parallel, and about a hip-width apart. Don't lean back—sit forward toward the front edge of the chair. Pull your head and shoulders back, and roll your hips forward and under into extension. You want an arch in your lower back. Your head, hips, and shoulders should be aligned and pointing straight at the ceiling. Interlace your fingers with the palms toward your stomach. Raise your arms, fingers still entwined straight over your head, and roll the palms of your hands toward the ceiling.

Figure 7.11

Tip your head back, and look upward at the back of your hands. Make sure your shoulders are back and the hips are still in extension. Don't shrug your shoulders. Your arms should be on either side of your head, lightly touching your ears. If they're not, and the head and ears are tipped back behind the arms, then your arms and upper body are not fully vertical; push your arms up and back. You'll feel your hips, lower back, and shoulders adjust and come into better alignment. Hold this position for thirty seconds. Remember to breathe, which will be difficult at first.

- STANDING QUAD
  STRETCH

This E-cise (figure
7.12) takes the
tension off the
secondary muscles
that flex the pelvis.
These muscles end up
doing double duty
when the primaries
are weakened by long
periods of being
hunkered down in a
chair.

Stand on one
foot, and bend the
other leg back,
placing the top of the
foot on a block, a
stool, or the back of a
chair. You'll want
about two and a half
feet of elevation,
although it depends

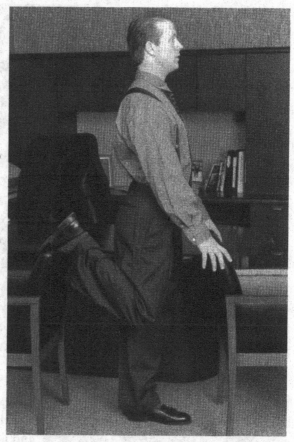

Figure 7.12

on how tall you are. The higher the block, the more stretch you'll feel in
the quadriceps. Keep your hips and shoulders square and your knees
even, and tuck your hips under to feel the stretch. (Roll them back to
create an arch in your back.) Hang on to something for balance. Hold
this position for one minute, then switch to the other side.

- SITTING CATS AND DOGS

This E-cise (figure 7.13a and b), like ordinary Cats and Dogs,
promotes mobility in the pelvis and back. Doing it while seated
provides the additional feature of loading the hip joints, which
encourages a vertical posture.

Sit in a chair with your feet flat on the floor, parallel, and about a hip-width apart. Don't lean back, but sit forward toward the front. Rest your hands palms-down by your thighs. Slowly pull your head, shoulders, and hips back into extension. Feel the arch in your lower back as your head moves back to the rear. Head, hips, and shoulders should be aligned and pointing straight at the ceiling (a). When you get there, pause for half a beat, and slowly relax, letting

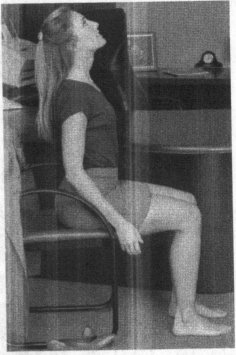

Figure 7.13a

Figure 7.13b

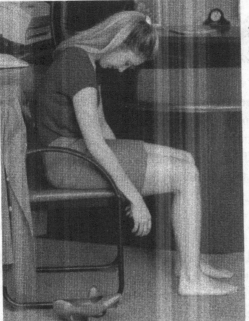

the back round forward and the shoulders, neck, and head come with it (b). We want the back to leave extension—but don't actually force your upper torso farther than its natural stopping point, where the muscles are fully relaxed. Link each Cat and Dog into a smooth, continuous series. Your hands will track back and forth on top of your thighs. Do ten. Remember to breathe.

• SITTING IN EXTENSION

This E-cise (figure 7.14) strengthens key posture muscles and reminds them what extension and proper alignment feel like. The more the posture muscles are put into this position, the better able they are to hold it on their own. If you can maintain this posture at the PC without deliberately thinking about it, there's little likelihood you'll ever experience computer pain syndrome. That's the alignment and function we're striving for with these E-cises.

Sit in a chair with your feet flat on the floor, parallel, and about a hip-width apart. Pull your head, shoulders, and hips back and into extension (arch your lower back). Breathe. Don't just yank your shoulders back or leave the head behind—head, shoulders, and hips must go together. Keep your feet in place. Balance the weight on both cheeks of your buttocks. Hold this position for one minute, and then relax.

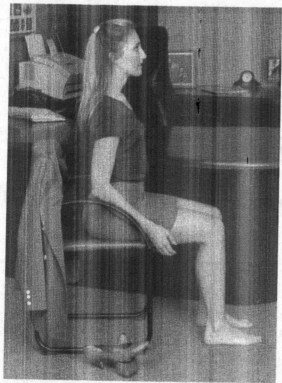

Figure 7.14

E-CISE MENU FOR MODERATE COMPUTER USERS

HOME THERAPY	OFFICE THERAPY
• Arm Circles	• Sitting in Extension
• Forearm Stretch	• Elbow Curls in Extension
• Wall Clock	• Sitting Assisted Hip Lift
• Static Back	• Three-Position Toe Raises
• Pullovers in Static Back	• Sitting Cats and Dogs
• Pullover Presses in Static Back	
• Cobra on Elbows	
• Supine Groin Stretch	
• Upper Spinal Floor Twist	
• Cats and Dogs	
• Air Bench	

The therapy in chapter 7 was designed for occasional PC users. I suspect, though, that eventually they will be a rare breed, and that the majority will fall into the category of moderate users. I'm probably being conservative. If PCs take over school classrooms—it's probably more realistic to say *when* they take over—and come anywhere close to matching TV as a popular medium, the vast majority of us will be power PC users. And that doesn't even take into account business applications.

We're not there yet, so by my definition a moderate PC user is someone who does not depend on a computer solely for his or her livelihood and uses one every day for about an hour in total. A good example would be a sales representative. He or she keeps her contacts on a PC or digital organizer, uses the computer for e-mail, and prepares proposals for customers. Maybe there's time for a video game. Occasionally a couple of back-to-back hours may be spent at the keyboard.

This extended PC use, while it may happen only once or twice a week, is a key reason for having this separate category. An hour or more of concentrated physical effort shouldn't be a big deal. But if I asked you to dig a hole for an hour without stopping, would it be taxing? Probably. And it would be particularly heavy going if you weren't used to doing that kind of work.

Why is that? For a moment forget about skeletal alignment and stability. The simple answer is that your muscles aren't strong enough. The same answer explains why a marathon run on the PC is also taxing. You're making thousands of contractions with muscles that otherwise, in the course of a day, contract only a few hundred times at most. Some hardly contract at all until they come to the PC. If you drive home from work for forty-five minutes, what are the muscles of your hands doing? Right—gripping the steering wheel. If you take the bus or the train, what are they doing? Holding a newspaper or a book, I'll bet.

The muscular effort was minimal in either case, compared with the PC. But as you know by now, simple muscular strength is not the primary issue. Dysfunctions are a wall standing between you and your primary muscles. The E-cises in this chapter restore access to these muscles and work on skeletal alignment and stability.

E-CISE TIPS

- Follow the menu in sequence.
- Don't pick and choose among E-cises. Do all of them in order.
- Honor the body's bilateral design by repeating the E-cises equally on both sides.
- Stop if the E-cise causes pain.
- Keep a slow, steady pace.
- Do at least one of the menus, home or office, once a day. Doing both would be ideal.
- If you miss a day or two, don't worry. Miss three or more—worry!
- On any given day, once you've run through the entire office therapy menu, feel free to take spontaneous E-cise breaks by choosing whichever one seems appropriate to the work you've been doing or the way your body is feeling.

Home Therapy Total Time: 40 minutes Frequency: Daily

• ARM CIRCLES

This E-cise is a ball-and-socket booster. Shoulder joints are bifunctional—they hinge forward and back, and they rotate in a ball-and-socket configuration. Using a mouse or keyboard means a lot of hinge demand, which often locks the shoulder in the forward position. This can happen in either the right or left shoulder—or both at the same time. Arm Circles counteract that tendency.

You may notice that each shoulder responds differently to this E-cise. This indicates that a bilateral structure has become unilateral. Don't favor one side or the other. In time they will strengthen and stabilize equally.

Stand with your head up, feet parallel about a hip-width apart, and arms at your sides. Curl the fingers of each hand into a light fist with your thumbs straight. (This is known as a "golfer's grip.") Raise your arms out to your sides, keeping the elbows and arms straight, palms down, and your thumbs pointing forward (a). Lift your arms until they are level with your shoulders. If one shoulder wants to pop up or swing forward, lower both until they stay level. (Pay attention to this, too, when you start doing the circles.) Now squeeze your shoulder blades together slightly, and rotate the arms forward in the direction the thumbs are pointing. Make a roughly six-inch-diameter circle. Keep your wrists and elbows straight—the

A.

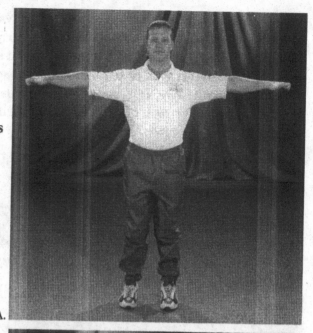

B.

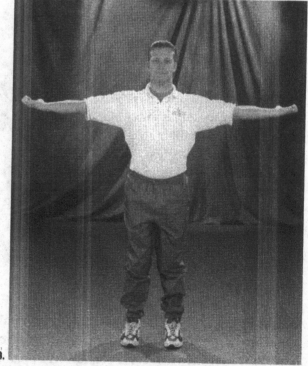

circles must come from the shoulders. Do this twenty-five times at a slow to moderate pace. Reverse the circles by turning the palms up and thumbs back (b). Crank the thumbs around so that your palms are level. Do another twenty-five. Then repeat back the other way for another twenty-five, and repeat again with the same count to the rear, so that you do a total of fifty in each direction. Remember to breathe.

• FOREARM STRETCH

This E-cise (figure 8.1) releases the tension in your wrists and forearms through the leverage provided by holding the shoulders in the correct position. Gradually you'll be able to position your hands higher on the wall, which should provide you with valuable information about the crucial interaction of the shoulders with the arms, forearms, wrists, and hands. You'll actually feel the interaction becoming less restricted and more complete.

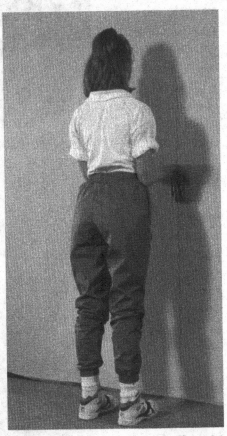

Figure 8.1

Facing a wall, stand with your feet straight and a hip-width apart. Your toes should be four to six inches from the wall. Bend your elbows to a ninety-degree angle, and place your palms against the wall with your fingers pointing down. Where you're able to place your hands will depend on the extent of shoulder function. The less you have, the lower they will be. If you feel wrist pain, lower your hands on the wall. If you can't find a hand position without wrist pain, you need to turn to chapter 6 and do the E-cise program there. Otherwise, lean against the wall with the weight on your hands, while squeezing your shoulder blades together. Make sure the heels of your palms are squarely on the wall. Don't shrug your shoulders or roll them toward the wall. They need to be back. Keep your stomach muscles relaxed, and allow the low back to arch. Hold for thirty seconds.

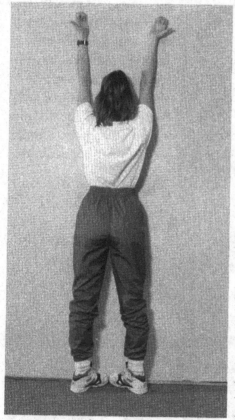

Figure 8.2a

• WALL CLOCK

Your shoulder blades are supposed to move—up and down, back and forth, and in clockwise and counter-clockwise rotation. When they don't, much of the dynamic relationship with the torso is lost, and much of the shoulders' biomechanical capacity is canceled out. This means that arm and hand movement at your PC's keyboard relies mostly on the elbow and wrist. This E-cise (figures 8.2a, b, and c) remedies that and releases the tension in the compensating muscles of your upper back and neck. The Wall Clock is a three-position E-cise.

Position one (a): Face the wall, and turn your feet inward in a pigeon-toed stance up against the wall. Raise your arms over your head in the twelve o'clock position. Your hands are gathered in a light fist with your thumbs straight, and the palms are facing each other. With your arms straight and still in

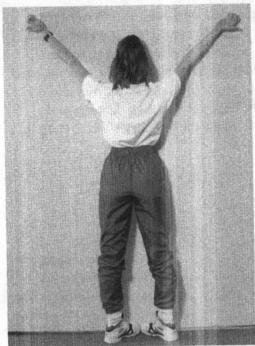

Figure 8.2b

contact with the wall, rotate your arms outward from the wall at your shoulders, with the thumbs flaring back at an angle from the wall. Hold this position for one minute.

Position two (b): Remain in the same pigeon-toed stance. Place your arms over your head in the ten-after-ten position. Your elbows are straight, while your shoulders are rotated away from the wall. The thumbs are pointing away from the wall. Hold for one minute.

Position three (c): Remain in the same stance. Place your arms over your head in the quarter-after-nine position. Your elbows are straight, while your shoulders are rotated away from the wall, with the thumbs pointing away from the wall.

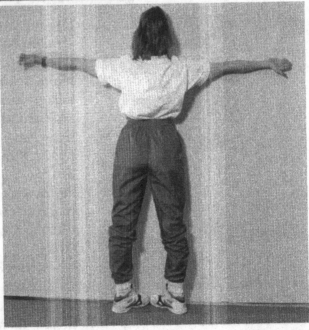

Figure 8.2c

Hold for one minute. If there is pain in your elbow in this position, you need to drop this menu and use the pain menu in chapter 6.

• STATIC BACK

This E-cise (figure 8.3) will settle the hips to the floor and allow the muscles of the upper torso to relax. Imagine what your hips are doing at the PC keyboard. Right—they are tipped back in flexion, instead of offering the spine a flat, neutral platform.

Lie on your back, with both legs bent at right angles resting on a chair or block. Rest your hands on your stomach or the floor, below shoulder level, with the palms up. Let the back settle into the floor. Breathe from your diaphragm. The abdominal muscles should rise as you inhale and fall as you exhale. Hold this position for five to ten minutes.

Figure 8.3

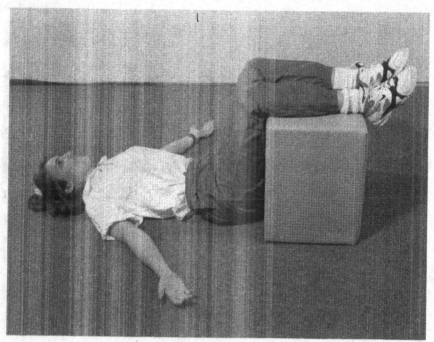

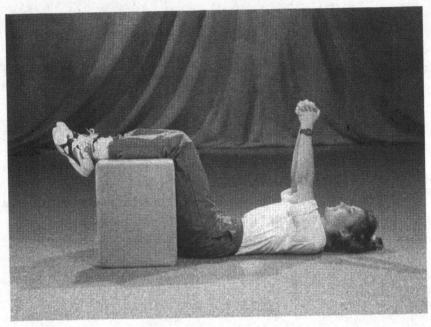

Figure 8.4a

Figure 8.4b

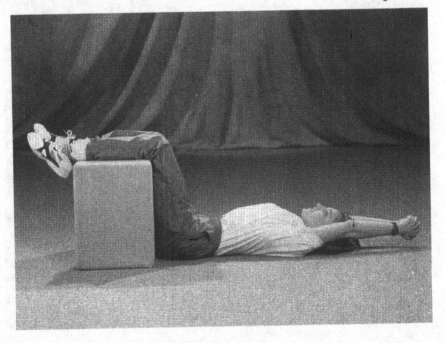

• Pullovers in Static Back

This E-cise (figures 8.4a and b) promotes the range of motion in your shoulders and releases the muscles of the neck and upper back. It also helps the diaphragm to work properly.

Stay in the basic Static Back position. Clasp your hands together, and extend your arms straight toward the ceiling (a). Continue to hold both arms straight, and bring them back behind your head, either to the floor or as far as they will go without bending (b). Then return to the starting position. Relax your abdominal muscles and don't rush. Do two sets of fifteen each.

• Pullover Presses in Static Back

This E-cise (figure 8.5) works to strengthen the muscles that hold the shoulder blades against the rib cage, instead of leaving them protracted.

Continue in the Static Back position. Place an eight-inch block

Figure 8.5

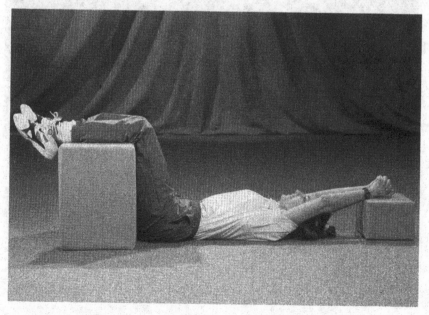

or a stack of books about an arm-length beyond your head. You'll want to be able to rest your hands squarely on the block during this E-cise. With hands clasped and arms straight, press and release into the block. Do not contract your abdominal muscles. Let your lower back muscles react, and keep your feet parallel. Do three sets of ten.

• COBRA ON ELBOWS

This E-cise (figure 8.6) strengthens the lower back muscles, releases tight abdominal muscles, and stabilizes the spine.

Lie on the floor on your stomach with your legs straight and your feet pigeon-toed. Use both elbows bent at ninety degrees to prop up the upper body. The elbows should be directly under the shoulder, the forearms straight and parallel. Make lightly clenched fists, with your thumbs pointing straight up. Your head looks straight ahead. Relax your buttocks muscles. Hold for thirty seconds.

Figure 8.6

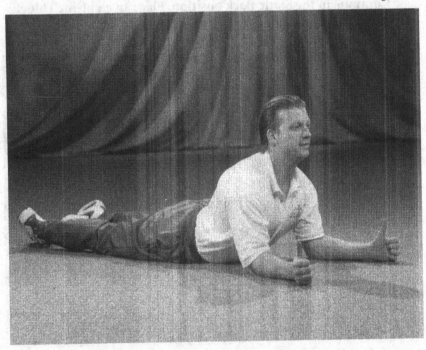

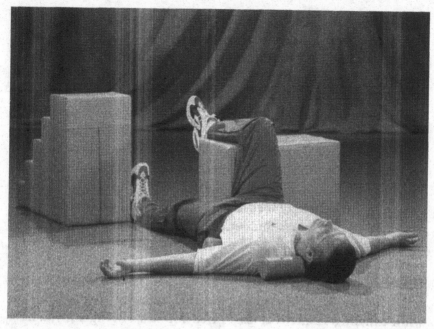

Figure 8.7

• SUPINE GROIN STRETCH

This E-cise (figure 8.7) relaxes and/or engages the primary muscles of hip flexion. It allows the pelvis to move into a neutral position, which isn't happening on its own.

Lie on your back, with one leg resting on a two-foot-high block or chair, the knee bent at a ninety-degree angle. The other leg is extended straight out and resting on the floor. Make sure both legs are aligned with the hips and shoulders. The foot of your extended leg should be propped upright to prevent it from rolling to one side. (Use something like a stack of books or a five-gallon paint can.) Relax in this position for at least ten minutes, then switch sides and remain for another ten minutes.

• UPPER SPINAL FLOOR TWIST

This E-cise can be a real eye-opener for people who don't think they have shoulder problems. One side will flatten to the floor readily, but the other may stay elevated. It means that one shoulder is having trouble returning to a neutral position.

Lie on your side with your knees together and bent. This will put your knees at a right angle to your trunk. Keeping the elbows straight and the palms together, extend both arms along the floor, level with your shoulders, in the direction of your knees, parallel with the bent legs. Slowly lift the upper arm up and over to rest behind you on the floor palm-up, while you turn your head to face the ceiling. Adjust this arm position, if necessary, by finding a shoulder slot that's comfortable. Relax and breathe deeply. Allow gravity to settle the extended arm to the floor along its entire length, from fingers to shoulder. Meanwhile, make sure the knees don't slide apart. You can hold them in place with the other hand (as the model is doing). When the shoulders have leveled out (it may take several minutes and perhaps several sessions to achieve this fully), lift the extended arm and return it to the starting position while exhaling. Hold for at least three minutes, or longer if you have the time and the shoulder hasn't come down onto the floor. Repeat on the other side.

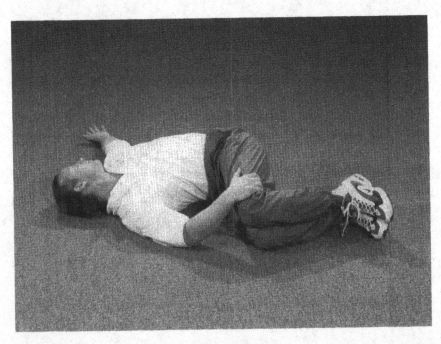

• CATS AND DOGS

This E-cise works you through cycles of flexion-extension from your hips to your head, providing total range of motion in the pelvis and the back in an anatomically correct and safe manner. It promotes breathing and better circulation. It's very effective, as you may know if you've done yoga.

Get down on the floor on your hands and knees. Make a "table" by aligning your hands under your shoulders and your knees and thighs under your hips. Your arms should be straight and your thighs parallel to them. Keep your legs and feet parallel to each other as well. The feet are relaxed and resting across the top side of the toes, not flexed or up on the toes. Make sure your weight is distributed evenly. Smoothly round your back upward as your head curls under, to create a curve that runs from the buttocks to the neck—this is a cat with an arched back (a). Smoothly sway the back down while bringing your head up—this is the perky dog (b). Make these two moves continuously back and forth—don't keep them choppy and distinct. Do one set of ten. Exhale as you

A.

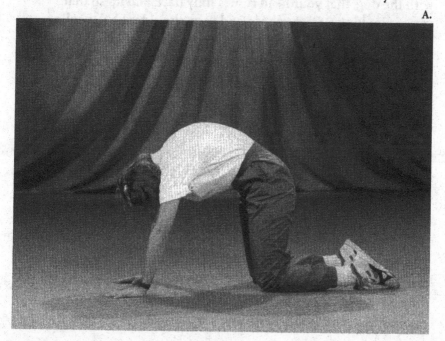

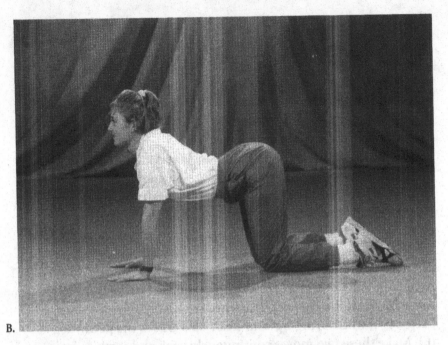

B.

move into the cat position, inhale during the dog. Make sure, with the dog, that your head comes fully back and up so that you are looking straight ahead and your shoulder blades collapse toward each other. Take your time. The pace should be slow, but not so slow that it breaks the flow between the cat and dog positions.

• AIR BENCH

This E-cise puts the ankles, lower legs, thighs, and hips to work in unison without relying on the back muscles for help. The Air Bench promotes lower-leg, thigh, and hip strength, and it relaxes the muscles of the torso. These are all functions we need to be pain free at the PC.

The best way to get into the starting position is to stand with your back to a wall. Press your hips and the small of your back into the wall. At the same time, walk your feet forward and simultaneously slip down the wall surface into a sitting position.

Stop when you've reached
approximately a ninety-degree
angle. Your knees should be
over your ankles, not your toes.
(You should be able to see your
toes.) If you feel pain in your
kneecaps, raise your body up
the wall to relieve the pressure.
Press the low back and midback
against the wall, and feel the
quadriceps working along the
tops of the thighs. Hold for
three minutes. Breathe. This
can be a struggle. You can
start by doing the Air Bench
for a few seconds and build to
a minute, extend it to two, and
then go for three. I've worked
with NFL running backs who
couldn't get beyond ten seconds
at first. When you are finished,
scoot back up the wall and walk
around for a few minutes.

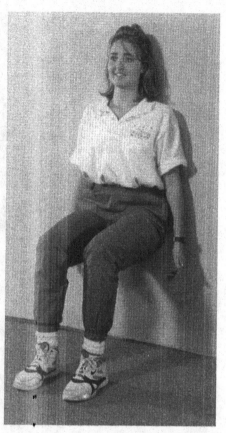

Office Therapy
Total Time: 5 minutes
Frequency: At least twice a week
Special Note: Remove your shoes

• SITTING IN EXTENSION

After the first few times, doing this E-cise will stop feeling strange,
and your vertical load-bearing muscles will get stronger and
stronger.

Sit in a chair with your feet flat on the floor, parallel, and about

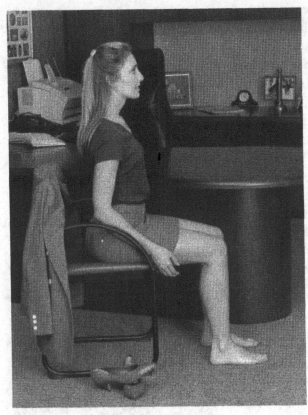

a hip-width apart. Pull your head, shoulders, and hips back and into extension (arch your lower back). Breathe. Don't just yank your shoulders back or leave the head behind—head, shoulders, and hips must go together. Keep your feet in place. Balance the weight on both cheeks of your buttocks. Hold the position for one minute, and then relax.

• ELBOW CURLS IN EXTENSION

This E-cise (figures 8.8a and b) releases the tight muscles of the lower back, thereby promoting range of motion in the shoulder and easing the tense muscles of the upper back and neck.

Sit in a chair. Move toward the front edge of the seat, away from the back. Set your feet flat on the floor, parallel, and a hip-width apart. Pull your head and shoulders back, while arching your back and rolling your hips forward into extension. Relax your stomach muscles, and breathe. Curl the fingers of both hands into a light fist with your thumbs straight. (This is known as the "golfer's grip.") Place the flat area formed between the first and second knuckle joints of the index and middle fingers on the temples in front of your ears; the thumbs extend downward, parallel with the cheeks.

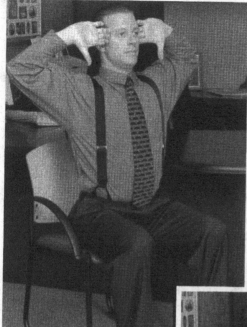

Figure 8.8a

Draw your elbows back evenly and in line with the shoulders (a). Don't allow one of them to be lazy and not come all the way back. Equalize the work and tension in both sides. From this starting position, slowly swing the elbows forward until they touch in front (b). Keep the knuckles in contact with the temples, the thumbs fully extended, and the

Figure 8.8b

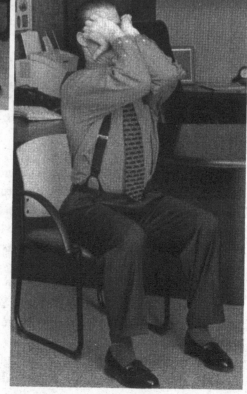

head erect. Don't let the hips or head wobble or seesaw. Breathe deeply. Do fifteen Elbow Curls.

- SITTING ASSISTED HIP LIFT

This E-cise (figure 8.9) activates external rotation of the femur (the thigh bone), thereby promoting

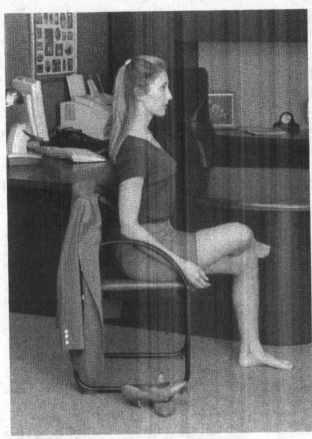

Figure 8.9

hip extension and relaxing the muscles of the lower back and torso. Through no fault of the PC, your hips may rotate right or left and stay that way. We need to give them the capacity to return to a balanced, symmetrical position.

Sit in a chair, toward the front edge of the seat. Your feet should be flat on the floor, parallel, and a hip-width apart. Pull your head and shoulders back, and roll your hips forward into extension. Imagine a vertical line extending through your hips, shoulders, and head to the ceiling. Bend your right leg, and place the ankle on your left knee. You may rest a hand on your bent right knee and use the other to help keep your right foot in place. Without pressing down with the hand, use the muscles of the thigh and hip area to draw your right bent knee toward the floor. Tighten the muscles slowly—you'll feel them pull the leg downward. Hold for thirty seconds. Repeat on the other side. You'll probably find that one side is tighter than the other and will give more resistance when you lower the knee.

Once you do both, return to the tighter side for another thirty seconds. You will have more downward play this time.

• THREE-POSITION TOE RAISES

This E-cise (figures 8.10a, b, and c) causes your pelvis to move into a neutral (planar) position while aligning the vertical load-bearing joints of the posture. We want the pelvis to sit flat, as if a shelf. It also runs both hips through the full flexion-neutral-extension cycle.

Position one (a): Near a closed door or wall, stand with your feet a hip-width apart and parallel. Pull your head and shoulders back, and roll the hips forward into extension to arch the lower back. Raise up on your toes, keeping your weight evenly distributed on both feet and your knees straight. Come straight up, don't rock

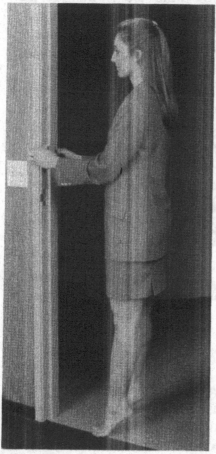

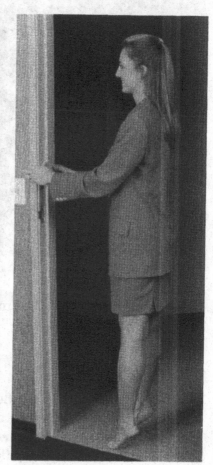

Figure 8.10a   Figure 8.10b

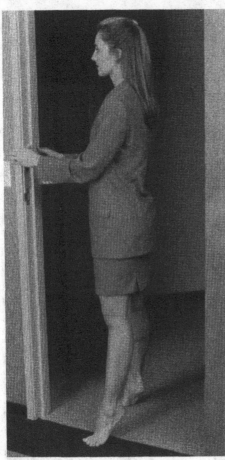

Figure 8.10c

forward. Make sure your weight isn't sloshing to the inside or outside of the feet; keep it even. Raise and lower yourself ten times.

Position two (b): Pull your head and shoulders back, and roll your hips forward into extension to arch the lower back. This time your feet should be pigeon-toed, with the big toes touching. Set the heels a hip-width apart, and angle your toes inward until they touch. Check the stance to make sure your weight is balanced between the two feet and distributed evenly over both feet. Keep the arch in your back. Raise and lower yourself ten times.

Position three (c): Stand in extension with your heels together and your feet spread like a duck with the toes pointed out. Raise and lower yourself ten times. Do these slowly to prevent your feet from rolling to the inner or outer edges.

• SITTING CATS AND DOGS

This E-cise works you through flexion and extension while your hips and torso are under a vertical load. But your hips, lower back, shoulders, and head must all participate.

Sit in a chair with your feet flat on the floor, parallel, and about a hip-width apart. Don't lean back, but sit forward toward the front.

Rest your hands palms-down by your thighs. Slowly pull your head, shoulders, and hips back into extension.

Feel the arch in your lower back as your head moves back to the rear. Head, hips, and shoulders should be aligned and pointing straight at the ceiling (a). When you get there, pause for half a beat, and slowly relax, letting the back round forward and the shoulders, neck, and head come with it (b). We want the back to leave extension—but don't actually force your upper torso farther than its natural stopping point, where the muscles are fully relaxed. Link each Cat and Dog into a smooth, continuous series. Your hands will track back and forth on top of your thighs. Do ten. Remember to breathe.

A.

B.

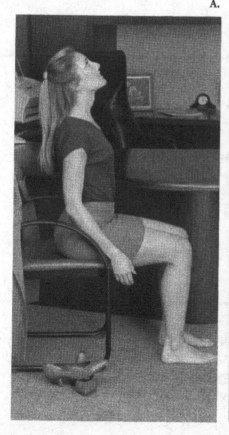
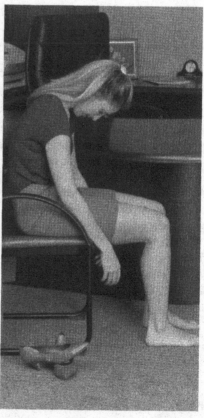

9

E-CISE MENU FOR POWER PC USERS

HOME THERAPY

- Static Back
- Abdominal Contractions in Static Back
- Abductor Presses in Static Back
- Standing Overhead Extension
- Elbow Curls at the Wall
- Static Wall with Pullbacks
- Static Extension Position
- Upper Spinal Floor Twist
- Pelvic Tilts
- Supine Groin Progressive
- Air Bench

OFFICE THERAPY

- Sitting in Extension
- Sitting Arm Circles
- Sitting Hip Flexor Lifts
- Sitting Chair Twist
- Sitting Cats and Dogs

Give me your hackers, your propeller-heads, your nerds, and all the rest of the *digerati* who know the difference between an ISP and an IPO (the IPO makes you rich, the ISP keeps you poor). Bring writers, editors, telemarketers, help desk personnel, designers, and all others who point, click, and type.

If you depend on the computer for your livelihood, this chapter is where you want to be for therapy. Timewise, I'm talking about using a PC for a minimum of more than an hour a day, every day. Is that all? Obviously, that's just the start. Six, eight, or ten hours a day may be closer to the norm for many people.

You are a member of the high-risk group. You're first to the future and in danger of being flummoxed by the pain. Not because the PC is dangerous—rather, you are living in a bubble of restricted movement for hour after hour. It's the reason why the total time for home therapy—and don't flip out!—is one hour and twenty minutes a day.

For those of you who haven't thrown this book across the room yet, that amount of time will quickly be whittled down to thirty minutes as you make progress with this E-cise program. The "time hog" that is part of this therapy program is the Supine Groin Progressive, an extremely effective E-cise for reestablishing your hips as a solid musculoskeletal foundation. But as the SGP takes hold, it needs less time. At first you'll have to invest in yourself. It's probably worth it—don't you think? There isn't much of an alternative if you want to remain on the cutting edge of the future.

E-CISE TIPS

- Follow the menu in sequence.
- Don't pick and choose among E-cises. Do all of them in order.
- Honor the body's bilateral design by repeating the E-cises equally on both sides.
- Stop if the E-cise causes pain.
- Keep a slow, steady pace.
- Do at least one of the menus, home or office, once a day. Doing both would be ideal.
- If you miss a day or two, don't worry. Miss three or more— worry!
- On any given day, once you've run through the entire office therapy menu, feel free to take spontaneous E-cise breaks by choosing whichever one seems appropriate to the work you've been doing or the way your body is feeling.

Home Therapy
Total Time: 1 hour and 20 minutes
Frequency: Daily

• STATIC BACK

By unloading the spine and hips, this E-cise uses gravity to relax your back muscles, which otherwise would remain in contraction and defeat the purpose of the next two strengthening E-cises. This E-cise will settle the hips to the floor and allow the muscles of the upper torso to relax. Imagine what your hips are doing at the PC keyboard. Right—they are tipped back in flexion, instead of offering the spine a flat, neutral platform.

Lie on your back, with both legs bent at right angles resting on a chair or block. Rest your hands on your stomach or the floor, below shoulder level, with the palms up. Let the back settle into the floor. Breathe from your diaphragm. The abdominal muscles should rise as you inhale and fall as you exhale. Hold this position for five to ten minutes.

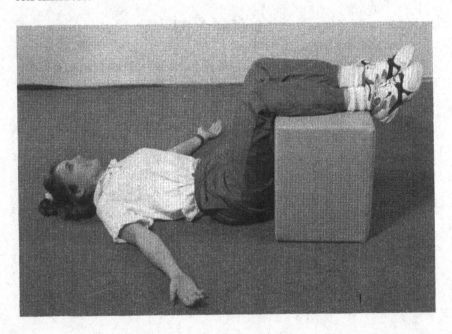

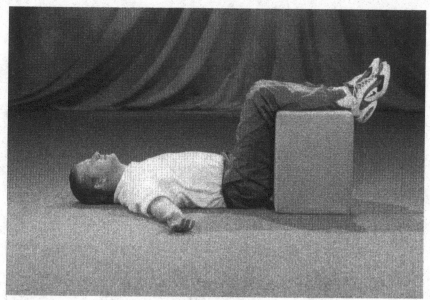

Figure 9.1

• Abdominal Contractions in Static Back

This E-cise (figure 9.1) promotes the use of the diaphragm and helps release the tight muscles in your trunk. We're teaching the body that you can have a flat stomach *and* breathe with your diaphragm, too. Most PC users roll forward at the keyboard, isolate their abs, and end up taking quick shallow breaths with their torso muscles, which operate only a small portion of the lungs.

In the Static Back position, inhale deeply and allow your stomach to rise. As you exhale, allow your stomach to fall. At the end of the exhalation, contract your abdominal muscles for a count of two and release. Repeat ten times.

• Abductor Presses in Static Back

This E-cise (figure 9.2) strengthens and releases the muscles of the pelvis that abduct the leg (that move it away from the center line), which promotes hip stability. You may notice as you do this menu

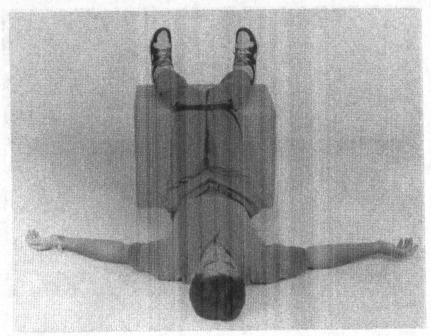

Figure 9.2

that you'll start to address the PC squarely, rather than scrunching to one side or the other. Abductor Presses to the rescue!

In the Static Back position, place a strap around your knees (just above the kneecaps on the thighs). Secure the strap so that your knees are together (touching), with the feet remaining a hip-width apart. Press outward against the strap, hold for one beat, and release. You should feel your hips doing the work. Keep your upper body relaxed. Do three sets of ten each.

• STANDING OVERHEAD EXTENSION

This E-cise (figure 9.3) opens up the thoracic back and the abdominal cavity, increases oxygen flow, and strengthens the muscles of extension in the back.

Stand with your feet parallel, a hip-width apart. Draw your head and shoulders back, and roll your hips forward into extension. You want an arch in your lower back. Interlace the fingers of your hands with the palms toward your stomach. Raise your arms, fingers still entwined, straight over your head, and roll the palms of your hands toward the ceiling. Make sure your shoulders are back and your hips still in extension. The arms should be on either side of the head, lightly touching the ears. Tip your head back and look upward at the back of your hands. Hold for thirty seconds. Remember to breathe, which will be difficult at first.

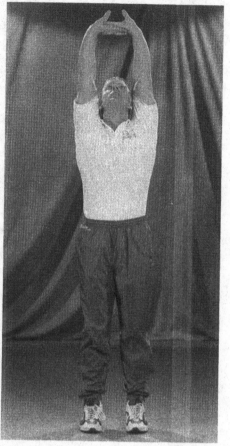

Figure 9.3

• ELBOW CURLS AT THE WALL

This E-cise eases the tension in the muscles of the upper back and neck, while promoting range of motion in the shoulder. Doing them against the wall prevents the head movement that will occur in people whose neck and shoulders are forward. I included it in the menu for light users in chapter 7, without the wall, because I've observed that most power PC users have so totally isolated their shoulder function that they cannot do Elbow Curls at first without a whole lot of head-shaking going on. Elvis wanted the hips to shake, not the head.

Stand with your back and head against a wall, with feet parallel and placed a hip-width apart. Put your hands in the golfer's grip, with fingers curled, knuckles flexed, and thumbs extended. Raise them palm-out so that the flat area on the backs of the index and middle fingers, between the first and second knuckle joints, rest on

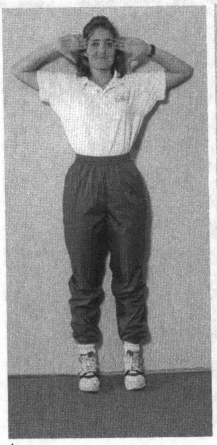

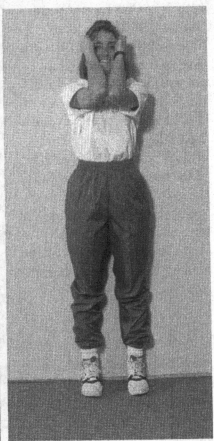

A.   B.

the temples in front of the ears; your thumbs extend downward,
parallel with your cheeks. Draw the elbows back evenly and in line
with the shoulders until both touch the wall (a). Don't allow one of
them to be lazy and not come all the way back. From this starting
position, slowly swing the elbows forward until they touch in front
(b). Keep the knuckles in contact with the temples, the thumbs fully
extended, and the head erect. Don't allow your head to wobble or
seesaw off the wall. Breathe deeply. Do twenty-five Elbow Curls.

• Static Wall with Pullbacks

This E-cise (figure 9.4) engages, strengthens, and stabilizes the hip.

Lie on your back at the foot of a wall. Place your legs straight up against the wall (so that your upper torso and legs are at ninety degrees), with your feet a hip-width apart. Tighten your thighs, and flex your toes and feet back toward the floor. Get your buttocks and hamstrings (the posterior of the thighs) as close to the wall as you can. The smaller the gap, the better. It may take several rounds of this E-cise to be able to get close to the wall. If your hips lift off the floor, back off until they are flat. Concentrate on relaxing your upper body. This is the Static Wall position.

For Pullbacks, with your thighs contracted, make sure your toes are flexed toward you and your legs are straight. Pull your right heel off the wall toward you by two or three inches, then return it to the wall. Do one set of fifteen. Repeat on the other side. You'll feel this in your thighs and hips.

Figure 9.4

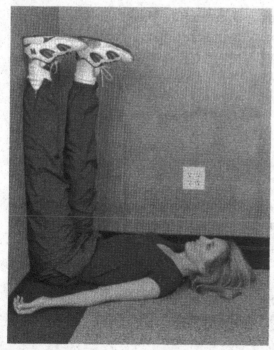

• Static Extension Position

This E-cise (figure 9.5) releases the contracted muscles in your trunk and builds strength in your hips. Try reading your e-mail from a notebook computer while doing this. I'm kidding, but it's not a bad idea.

Get down on the floor on your hands and knees. Your hands should be about six inches forward of your

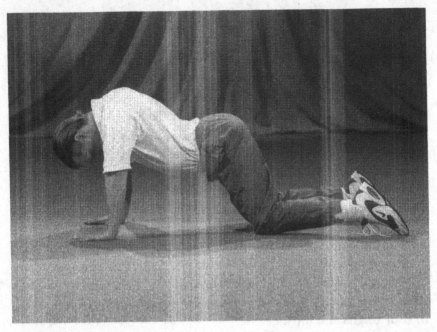

Figure 9.5

shoulders to start, rather than directly under them. Let your back and head relax toward the floor as the shoulder blades come together. Relax. There should be a pronounced arch in your back. Keep your arms straight, and shift your hips forward six to eight inches so that they are not aligned with the knees. This will also bring your shoulders into line over your wrists. Hold for one to two minutes.

● UPPER SPINAL FLOOR TWIST

Having released your contracted shoulder and upper torso muscles with the last E-cise, this one restores full range of motion to the shoulders.

Lie on your side with your knees together and bent. This will put your knees at a right angle to your trunk. Keeping the elbows straight and the palms together, extend both arms along the floor, level with your shoulders, in the direction of your knees, parallel with the bent legs. Slowly lift the upper arm up and over to rest

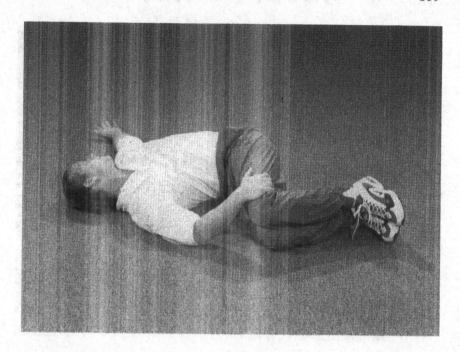

behind you on the floor palm-up, while you turn your head to face
the ceiling. Adjust this arm position, if necessary, by finding a
shoulder slot that's comfortable. Relax and breathe deeply. Allow
gravity to settle the extended arm to the floor along its entire
length, from fingers to shoulder. Meanwhile, make sure the knees
don't slide apart. You can hold them in place with the other hand
(as the model is doing). When the shoulders have leveled out (it may
take several minutes and perhaps several sessions to achieve this
fully), lift the extended arm and return it to the starting position
while exhaling. Hold for at least three minutes, or longer if you have
the time and the shoulder hasn't come down onto the floor. Repeat
on the other side.

● PELVIC TILTS

This E-cise strengthens and releases the muscles of the torso.
    Lie on your back with your knees bent, your feet flat on the
floor, and your hands resting at your sides, palms up. Roll your hips

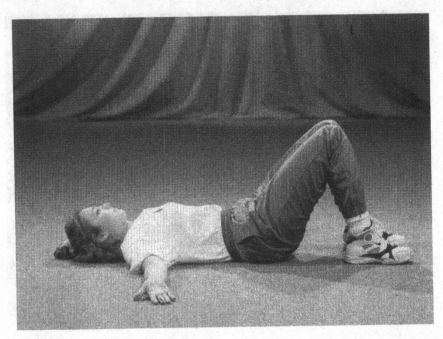

A.

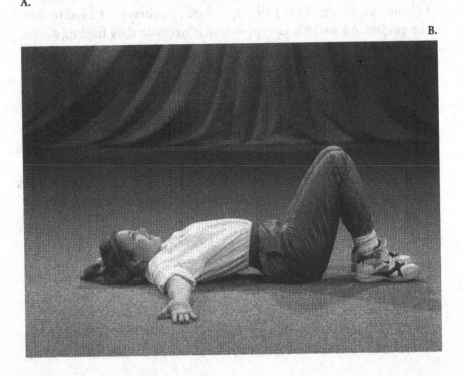

B.

toward your head to flatten your lower back into the floor (a). Do not lift your hips off the floor. Then roll your hips away to make the lower back arch off the floor, creating a space between the floor and your back (b). Do these rolls in a smooth continuous motion as you flatten and arch the back. Remember to breathe in sync with the hip movement—inhale up, exhale down. Do ten tilts. Don't move your feet or flap your knees.

• SUPINE GROIN PROGRESSIVE

This E-cise (figure 9.6) unlocks tight hip flexor muscles, which keep the pelvis tipped down to the rear in the flexion position. It is one of the most effective dysfunction-busters for a power PC user who spends hours sitting with his or her hips cranked into flexion.

You need a two-foot block, bench, or chair without arms. Also obtain a stepladder, shelving, or a cabinet with drawers that can be

Figure 9.6

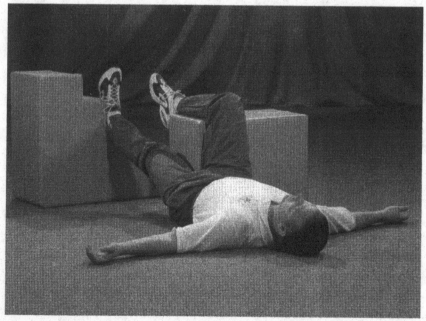

pulled open to function like the apparatus we use in the clinic. What's required is something that steps down from fifteen inches to ten, to five, and to the floor. Lie on your back with one leg resting on the chair or block; bend the knee at a ninety-degree angle, and let the foot hang over the edge unsupported. Extend the other leg straight, and place the heel of the foot on the fifteen-inch rung of the ladder. (You can also start at ten.) Use a book or another heavy object to brace the foot in an upright position; otherwise it will want to roll outward. Hold this position for at least ten minutes. Lower the foot to the next level down, and hold for another ten minutes. Lower the foot to the next level (or to the floor, if you started at ten inches), and hold for ten minutes. Switch legs and repeat on the other side. Breathe from your diaphragm. Relax.

This E-cise is time-consuming but worth it. The ideal way to determine when you are ready to drop to the next level is to contract your thigh muscles. If there is a solid contraction in the middle of the thigh, about halfway between the hip and the knee, you are ready to lower the leg. You are not ready if the knee or hip jerks or twitches when the thigh muscles contract. Overall, what you are looking for is a relaxation and release of tension from the ankle to the groin. The more you do this E-cise, the less time it takes. Eventually, a couple of minutes at each level will be enough. Getting to that point may take anywhere from one month to over a year, depending on how entrenched your dysfunctions are. In the process, though, it's a great way to watch TV or listen to music.

● AIR BENCH

This is a team-building E-cise. Your hips, knees, and ankles need to practice working together while the major muscle groups are under contraction. The Air Bench promotes lower-leg, thigh, and hip strength, and it relaxes the muscles of the torso. These are all functions we need to be pain free at the PC.

The best way to get into the starting position is to stand with your back to a wall. Press your hips and the small of your back into

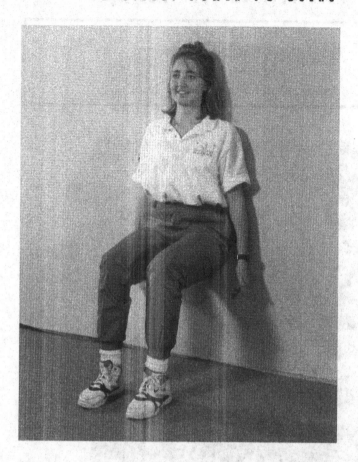

the wall. At the same time, walk your feet forward and simultaneously slip down the wall surface into a sitting position. Stop when you've reached approximately a ninety-degree angle. Your knees should be over your ankles, not your toes. (You should be able to see your toes.) If you feel pain in your kneecaps, raise your body up the wall to relieve the pressure. Press the low back and midback against the wall, and feel the quadriceps working along the tops of the thighs. Hold for three minutes. Breathe. This can be a struggle. You can start by doing the Air Bench for a few seconds and build to a minute, extend it to two, and then go for three. I've worked with NFL running backs who couldn't get beyond ten seconds at first. When you are finished, scoot back up the wall and walk around for a few minutes.

> Office Therapy
> Total Time: 5 minutes
> Frequency: Daily
> Special Note: Remove your shoes

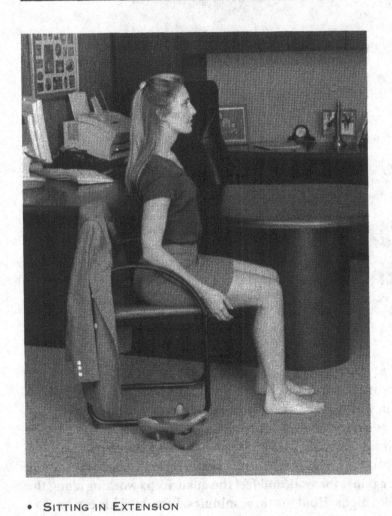

• SITTING IN EXTENSION

Do this E-cise enough, and you won't need or want a fancy desk chair.

Sit in a chair with your feet flat on the floor, parallel, and about a hip-width apart. Pull your head, shoulders, and hips back and into extension (arch your lower back). Breathe. Don't just yank your shoulders back or leave the head behind—head, shoulders, and hips must go together. Keep your feet in place. Balance the weight on both cheeks of your buttocks. Hold this position for one minute, and then relax.

• SITTING ARM CIRCLES

This E-cise (figures 9.7a and b) promotes hip extension and strengthens the muscles of the upper body.

Sit toward the front edge of a chair, with your head and shoulders back and your hips rolled forward in extension; your feet are squared about a hip-width apart, and your arms are at your sides. Put your hands in the golfer's grip, with fingers curled, knuckles flexed, and thumbs extended. Raise your arms out to your sides, keeping the elbows straight, palms down, and thumbs pointing forward (a). Lift your arms until they are level with your shoulders. If one shoulder wants to pop up or swing forward, lower both until they stay level. (Pay attention to this, too, when you start doing the circles.) Now squeeze the shoulder blades together slightly, and rotate the arms forward in the direction the thumbs are pointing. Make a roughly six-inch-diameter circle.

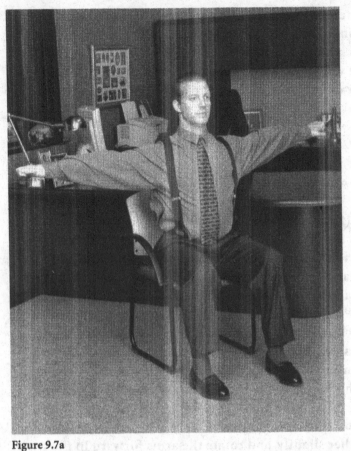

Figure 9.7a

Keep the elbows straight—the rotation must be in the shoulders. Do it twenty-five times. Reverse the circles by turning the palms up and thumbs back (b). Do another twenty-five. Then repeat back the other way for another twenty-five, and repeat again with the same count to the rear, so that you do a total of fifty in each direction.

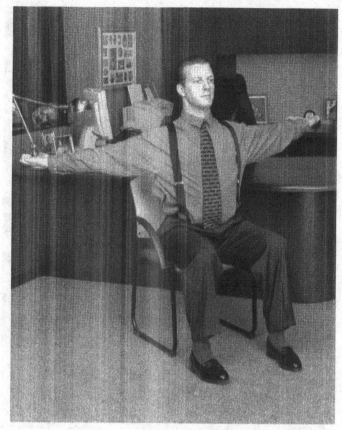

Figure 9.7b

• Sitting Hip Flexor Lifts

This E-cise (figure 9.8) is red meat for your hip flexor muscles. It is a deceptively simple strengthening routine.

Sit toward the front edge of a chair, with your head and shoulders back, your arms at your sides, and your hips rolled forward into extension; your feet are parallel and a hip-width apart. Keep your weight evenly balanced on both cheeks of the buttocks. Lift your right foot about an inch off the floor, using your thigh muscles. Hold it a half beat, and lower it. Do this ten times. Switch

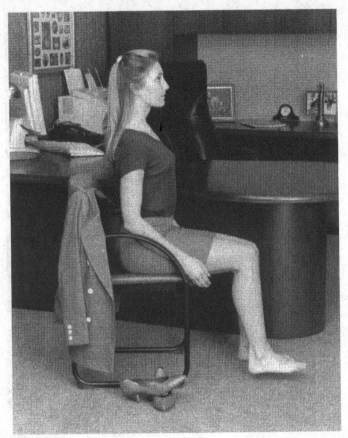

Figure 9.8

to the other leg for another count of ten. Make sure you don't lean to the side or lift with the hips. Keep the lift to an inch or less, otherwise the thigh muscles will be bypassed.

• SITTING CHAIR TWIST

This E-cise (figure 9.9) promotes trunk stability by strengthening those muscles and releasing tension. Your PC is never going to demand bilateral hip and trunk rotation. It's happy if you just sit there with little or no rotation at all. Problems occur when you get up and need the rotation for other purposes—like backing the car out its parking space.

This works best in a chair with arms. Sit with your feet on the floor, parallel, and a hip-width apart. Pull your head and shoulders back, and roll your hips forward into extension. Rotate your upper body to the right by grasping the right arm of the chair with your left hand. Bend your right arm over the chair back to grasp its left edge or the other arm. Keep your head level, and don't let your knees spread farther apart. Don't shrug your shoulders. Hold this position for twenty to thirty seconds. Breathe. Repeat on the left side.

Figure 9.9

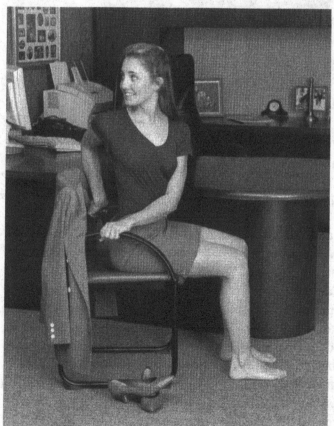

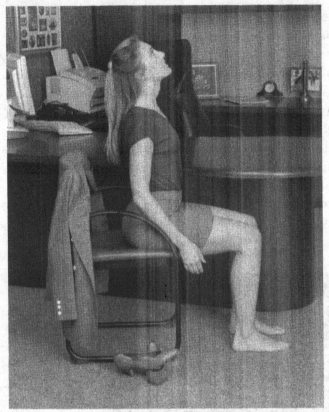

A.

• SITTING CATS AND DOGS

This E-cise is about as close as you can come to a do-it-yourself back massage. But not only does it feel good, it strengthens muscles and functions.

Sit in a chair with your feet flat on the floor, parallel, and about a hip-width apart. Don't lean back, but sit forward toward the front. Rest your hands palms-down by your thighs. Slowly pull your head, shoulders, and hips back into extension. Feel the arch in your lower back as your head moves back to the rear. Head, hips, and shoulders should be aligned and pointing straight at the ceiling (a). When you get there, pause for half a beat, and slowly relax, letting the back round forward and the shoulders, neck, and head come with it (b).

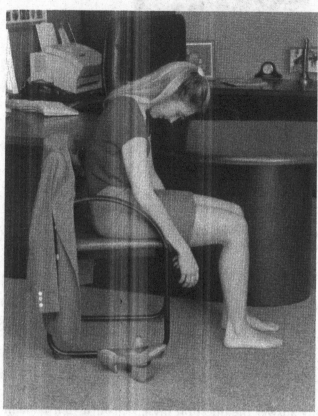

B.

We want the back to leave extension—but don't actually force your
upper torso farther than its natural stopping point, where the
muscles are fully relaxed. Link each Cat and Dog into a smooth,
continuous series. Do ten. Remember to breathe.

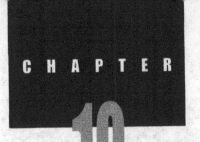

CHAPTER 10

OTHER SYMPTOMS, OTHER CHOICES

"When you're working at the PC, your eyes are as busy as your hands, wrists, and arms."

Pain is a powerful motivator. It's probably the main reason you bought this book. But what if you had been in no pain or there was only a remote possibility that a painful condition might arise?

I can probably answer the question myself: *Spotted your tome in the bookstore, Pete, but bought a copy of* Using Visual C+++ Basic$_6$ *instead.*

Okay, I understand. Human nature is human nature. *You* should understand, though, that symptoms of underlying musculoskeletal dysfunction can be present even when pain is absent. The E-cises in chapters 6, 7, 8, and 9 address them effectively, but not—*not*—if you decide that since the pain's gone, it's pointless to continue with the E-cises.

When pain abates, many people play what I call *pain-pong:* It hurts—they do something—it stops hurting. They go back to business as usual, until it starts to hurt again. They do something, it stops hurting, and . . . on and on. With each cycle there is more damage and a steeper recovery curve to climb. Eventually, the pain settles in and becomes chronic.

I don't want you to play pain-pong. In this chapter and those that follow, I'm going to try and provide you with some continuing motivation, starting with good old-fashioned fear.

What is pain? Pain is a *next*-to-last-resort symptom. Paralysis comes next. The final stop is death.

Whoa!

I am absolutely serious. Pain is the highest form of communication that the body possesses. When it occurs, a priority message is being sent. One of the reasons that the body resorts to this rude attention-grabbing device is that we've ignored other messages that came in more genteel forms. Skeletal misalignment, for instance, is a way to notify us that something is wrong. Long before a muscle pulls or a joint swells, there is an outward visible sign—a symptom—of illness. Catch it at that stage, and there's no problem. Wait until there's damage, however, and the slide to paralysis begins.

Not long ago, I was running behind a twentysomething woman beside the railroad track that stretches along the bluff above the Pacific Ocean near my home in California. It's a spectacular place for a workout, but I was looking at her rather than at the view. She seemed very fit, yet as she ran, her knees were tracking inward instead of pushing through flexion and extension directly over her feet. It was as if she were running knock-kneed. This is a common condition, known as valgus stress. The body's weight is being projected to the inside of the knees and ankle joints. As a result the design of all these structures is seriously impaired. The shock of the foot's impact is not being absorbed squarely by either the knees or by the ankles; as they open and close, a violent torquing or lateral twisting is occurring in the joint capsules.

KNEE KNOWLEDGE

A functional knee "looks" in the direction that the feet are pointing. To see how functional yours are, stand facing a full-length mirror with your feet pointed straight ahead. (Wear a pair of shorts so you can see your knees.) If the kneecap(s) squints or scrunches off to the left or right, it means your femur, the thigh bone, is being twisted and repositioned in the hip socket. This symptom of joint misalignment explains why many people with wrist and shoulder pain also have problems with their knees and ankles. It confirms how interrelated the body is from head to toe.

Valgus stress is a symptom. In the runner's case, it's a symptom of a broken ankle. She doesn't know it, but in a week, a month, a year, five years, she will step out of the shower or off the curb and break an ankle. Maybe her knee will blow first. Either way, she is a casualty-in-waiting. The symptom is there. Once the accident happens, her days of serious running are over. There may be other recreational activities—biking or in-line skating—yet over time there will be a pattern of less and less motion.

This gradual dwindling of motion can be deceptive. The body is so strong and so innately apprehensive of immobility that it's able to adjust downward by making small sacrifices of functional movement on the assumption that the motion deficit will eventually be corrected. The decline happens gradually; it fools us into thinking we are "aging" or making lifestyle choices or that we are "too busy." Worse, we don't even notice this slide. With the loss of vertical load-bearing, little by little we forfeit our unhindered capacity to move. Incrementally, it drains away. Pain comes and goes, as do other symptoms. Discomfort sets in, accidents happen. One day there is a major event like a stroke or heart attack.

This death spiral is sobering, but its logic should give us great hope. Instead of quickly flipping a switch and shutting down, the body buys time to allow corrective action. Until very late in the game, intervention can have dramatically positive results. My objective here is to call these nonpain symptoms to your attention. Then you can take action. Better yet, the action is already an ongoing process.

The Eyes Have It

There are estimates that 80 percent of regular PC users complain of eyestrain, eye fatigue, burning, blurring, and what have you. A good reason to continue the E-cises is that they are all working to counteract these conditions by restoring ocular muscular functions and the musculoskeletal structures that support them. Let me show you what I mean.

Take a deep breath.

Deeper.

And another.

AIR RAID

The diaphragm is a large, flat, shelflike muscle that sits under the lungs. By contracting and relaxing, it pumps air in and out of the lungs. As we lose vertical load-bearing, with the head, shoulders, and rib cage moving forward and down, the diaphragm is being constricted by the structures of the thoracic and abdominal cavities. This is a major impediment to oxygen intake, which makes it more difficult for our muscles to function properly. Given the intense muscular activity in the eye, which is burning up energy at a high rate, the eyes are quick to feel this oxygen deprivation.

You just fed your muscles and the rest of the body's tissue. All muscles, large and small, are acutely dependent on blood flow and the oxygen it delivers. Furthermore, when they are healthy and fully functional, these muscles are all instrumental in facilitating the delivery of oxygen throughout the body; some, like the diaphragm, are direct participants, while others work indirectly. Funny thing about that—somehow the lungs just don't inhale and exhale on their own.

Another funny thing: A muscle that makes few contractions is using commensurably less energy than one that makes many contractions. It seems obvious, but our big, showy muscles are not necessarily the major consumers of the body's store of energy. Although relatively small, the ocular muscles, as they focus and scan, are among the body's most active muscles. When you're working at the PC, your eyes are as busy as your hands, wrists, and arms. In addition, the optic nerve uses more oxygen than any other nerve in the body. This means eyes have a huge appetite for oxygen. Nonetheless, eye muscles experience the same ill effects of skeletal misalignment and resulting muscular dysfunction as our major posture muscles and prime movers.

The poets say the eye is the window of the soul. If you know what to look for when you peer into those windows, you can see a hell of a fight going on. Muscles that are located in the skull—jaw, eyes, nose, and ears—are caught in the middle of a war zone. Two other "armies" are fighting for a limited supply of oxygen. These more powerful forces are the brain and the muscles of the cervical spine—the section between the shoulders and the base of the skull. The power comes from desperation.

The brain always dominates. It lays immediate claim to the largest share of the oxygen flow, and it will use the central nervous system to ruthlessly curtail other functions to get what it needs. Meanwhile, the cervical spine is struggling frantically with a major concern of its own. With the loss of vertical load-bearing, the head moves forward and down, and the cervical spine must fend off gravity to keep the head upright.

By design, as the spinal column ascends, it gets slimmer and more flexible. This is a sensible arrangement, since there's no longer an involvement in major upper-torso functions, such as hefting the more massive thoracic back and shoulder girdle. There's less surface area, however, for flexion and extension. DROM, design range of motion, did not foresee the need to counterbalance eight to ten pounds of skull that wants to roll south. Nor did DROM figure on hip flexion reshaping the spine's S-curve into a C. Hence, to keep the head upright, the overwhelmed neck muscles start locking into flexion. A contracted muscle is like an open spigot: energy spews through it wildly to maintain contraction.

See the problem? Between the greedy brain and the desperate neck muscles, the muscles of the eye are being run dry. With the E-cises that have been presented, we're helping to reposition the hips and allow the cervical spine to release from flexion. We're turning off the spigot.

Not only does that decrease the demand for energy from the neck area, but the muscles can resume participating in their role of aiding the uphill flow of blood to the skull as they mechanically contract-relax-contract in flexion and extension adjacent to the arteries carrying the blood.

At the same time, as the S-curve of the spine is restored, lung capacity increases because the upper body is no longer collapsing down on the diaphragm. There's generally more oxygen in circulation. Our underlying metabolic rate picks up, which reinvigorates all the body's tissues and functions.

As the neck recovers its proper function, you may notice that another nonpain symptom abates. Your head will begin to be able to turn more easily to the left and right. To look over our shoulders, we need to be able to access shoulder muscles and functions. A neck frozen in contraction can't do that. Have you had a few fender benders lately, or near misses when changing lanes?

Hindsight About Far Sight

We already discussed how the body suspends muscles and functions it doesn't use. Just for the sake of consistency, doesn't it make sense for underutilized eye functions to also be put on hold? There's strong evidence that native peoples, American Indians, Australian Aborigines, and others who predate so-called civilization rarely developed routine vision problems. The probable reason for this helps explain what's happening with your eyes in front of the PC.

Whether they were indigenous fishers and hunters of the arctic circle or nomadic desert foragers and herders, a common phrase in their separate languages roughly translates to "He who looks far." To survive day by day, those people used their eyes to "look far." Today we look close. Most of our work is done at less than arm's length. Functions that provide us with extended vision are rarely accessed.

What we no longer use, we lose. Try to remember the last time you really focused on a distant point on the horizon. Compare that one

---

EYES: GOING THE DISTANCE

- Choose an object in the far distance, another in the middle, and one up close. You should be able to focus on them by shifting your eyes without changing the head position. Now, look at the far object, and bring it into focus as sharply as you can. Once focus is achieved, switch to the middle object without moving your head. Focus again. Finally, shift to the nearest object, and *take as long as you need* to bring it into focus. Again, don't shift your head position. Repeat the cycle by shifting back to the distant object.

- Do this twenty times, twice a day. At first you will notice that your eyes are really working hard to achieve focus. There will be a different feel in each zone. Gradually it will become easier and more uniform. Also, if you pay attention to the time it takes to focus on the close object, you'll discover that this will become much quicker to lock in.

- Burning, blurring, and eye fatigue should start to improve in about two weeks. Check with your eye doctor to make sure there aren't other underlying conditions like diabetes or high blood pressure.

event to the number of close-ups that occur. The ratio is enormously unbalanced. Extended vision for many people amounts to looking down the highway by one or two car lengths (or less!). But you may wonder, "If extended vision is being lost, why am I having fatigue when I use my eyes for close work on the PC?"

The answer is that the two functions work together and mutually support each other. Compromise one, and the other is affected. Likewise, you can strengthen the whole unit. The exercise on page 127 is one we use in the clinic to help people with headaches and vision problems.

Headaches are also incorrectly blamed on PCs. Here again, oxygen deprivation is at work. As with eyestrain, restoring vertical alignment and musculoskeletal function is the key to getting relief. The most common forms of headaches are the result of nerve fibers at the base of the skull, in the scalp, and on the face being impinged by dilated blood vessels that are under stress from oxygen loss and are reacting to intense muscular contractions in the neck. All the E-cise programs serve as quick oxygen boosters.

When I was a teenager, my mother was a migraine sufferer. She used to lie down in a dark room with wet towels over her eyes. It was one of the only things that would relieve the pain. As the moisture in the towels condensed and cooled, it induced the capillaries, which had increased their normal surface areas in order to soak up as much scarce oxygen as possible, to shrink again. It worked—temporarily. Before long, though, once my mother got back on her feet, the continued lack of oxygen would start to bedevil the blood vessels again. The terrible cycle would repeat itself. Today I'd urge her to use the E-cises to release the contracted muscles in her cervical and thoracic spinal curves.

Water Works

Those who experience frequent migraines and other less intense forms of headaches share a common nonpain symptom with many PC users—dehydration. Lack of motion and the musculoskeletal dysfunctions that result disrupt the body's metabolic processes. When we don't

ON THE BLINK

I could tell when my friend Adrien was getting really successful with his Internet startup company: He stopped moving and blinking. He sits in meetings or on the telephone all day instead of hustling to round up business. The last time we met, I asked him, "Are your eyes bothering you?"

"How did you know? They burn something awful."

I told him that he had hardly blinked at all in forty-five minutes. Adrien was dehydrated.

The eye lubricates itself by blinking. When there is no natural moisture, the blink rate falls off. A dry eyelid is irritating and might abrade the eyeball. If your eyes are dry or burning, like Adrien's, it may be a symptom of success.

fuel the body properly, it literally starts running dry. Perversely, our survival instinct and mechanisms make matters worse. Sensing that there is a drought, the body switches off the desire for water to help get us through the crisis. The less water we drink, the less we think we need to drink.

The drought keeps getting worse. The less we drink, the less we move. The less we move, the more we undermine the metabolic process. Your E-cise program will counter that if you focus on what your body is telling you, as opposed to what your habits are saying. Metabolism aside, you are probably out of the habit of drinking enough water to hydrate your system. The E-cises will make you thirsty again, but habit will try to distract you.

"I don't drink water."

"I don't like water."

"I prefer cola."

"Water goes through me too fast, and I have to pee every ten minutes."

Name the excuse, and I've heard it. I can stroll through any Silicon Valley firm, and what I will see are the accoutrements of pain: cola cans and coffee cups, sugary fruit potions, and the megacaffeine drinks that Gen-Xers love to binge on; plus candy, potato chips, and other salty snacks. What we are trying to do with these sweet beverages and sodium-laden starches is to jolt the system and get it back up to speed.

The temporary blast from the salt, sugar, or caffeine wears off quickly. Furthermore, by messing with your blood sugar levels, it tricks your system into assuming that the body has been properly and nutritionally refueled—*Where else would the extra sugar be coming from, if*

A LIQUID E-CISE

With your right or left hand, grasp a large drinking cup (10–12 ounces). Fill this container with water from a filtered system or a bottle of still spring water. (Carbonation is gas and it's competing with oxygen.) Start with the elbow held at ninety degrees, and slowly raise the forearm, hand, and cup to the lips. Drink. Do this throughout the day to consume at least ten full cups. There will be an additional motion dividend in the trips you take back and forth to the bathroom. Enjoy the walk!

not from carbohydrates? Thus, the sugar is stored as fat, while the more accessible muscle tissue is burned off for energy.

Now, in this horror scenario, do you see three more nonpain symptoms? I do: obesity, high blood pressure, and fatigue. The last two are natural by-products of a system that is struggling to make do with fewer and fewer resources. It's hard not to be fatigued when the metabolic process can't deliver the energy we need. And being "overweight" is usually the definition of obesity, but a more accurate standard is a disproportionate ratio of fat to muscle. This manifests itself in a body type that seems prevalent among serious male PC users—sorry, guys— a small and growing paunch on an otherwise lean frame. You might call this "slimbesity" as opposed to obesity: With the upper and lower extremities disengaged, muscle mass and definition are receding toward the abdomen and hips.

That physique is a nonpain symptom, too. It has very little to do with genetics. And it certainly has nothing to do with computers. PCs will surely change our lives, but we are the ones who are transforming our bodies from *motion-full* to *motion-less*.

CHAPTER 11

BREAKING THE PATTERNS OF PAIN

"Modern life is increasingly conducted inside of an invisible box floating directly in front of you that covers an area from about midthigh to the shoulders."

During the Vietnam war, American POWs were often punished by their North Vietnamese jailers by being confined to tiny "tiger cages" that were about four feet wide, four feet deep, and five feet high. The prisoners sat there for days and weeks at a time. When they were released, these brave men could hardly crawl.

Today you may spend days and weeks confined to a similar-size cage called a "computer workstation." Imagine the space that you usually work in delineated by bars or cold cement walls. I'm not talking about a cubicle or tiny office—those are bad in their own right. I'm interested in that bit of real estate that holds your keyboard, screen, mouse, and chair. If you were, in fact, sealed off from the rest of the world, it would be psychologically intolerable. But when the walls are invisible, there is an illusion of space that is comforting. I want you to start thinking like a prisoner and begin planning how to escape.

It's not necessary to quit your job or junk the PC. Just open the door and let yourself out of jail from time to time.

The object is to break the patterns of restricted motion that have become habitual or those that seem to be dictated by technology and work requirements. This is no easy task. We're conditioned to take motion for granted. And why wouldn't we? It happened naturally for

ESCAPISM

- Move the wastebasket to a different spot every day (never within easy reach).
- Place the phone console on the far side of your desk.
- If you are right-handed, answer the phone with your left hand.
- Never use a telephone headset (if you can help it).
- When possible, take calls standing up.
- When put on hold, inhale and exhale deeply using your diaphragm for the duration of the wait.
- Make it a point to stand when a colleague enters your work area to conduct a conversation.
- Stand up at the end of each discrete task.
- Change the height of your desk chair every day.
- Switch your style of desk chair each week (and the less chair the better).
- Change your monitor position each morning and afternoon.
- Raise or lower your keyboard daily.
- Place working materials and references on the floor so that you must bend over to get them.
- Rearrange the furniture in your work area once a month.
- Place frequently used material on the top shelf of a tall book-case.
- Place frequently used material on the bottom shelf of a book-case.
- Use a rest room that is upstairs, downstairs, or in an inconvenient spot.
- Take a walk for half your lunch hour, or go to the gym to work out.
- When the boss isn't looking, lean back and put your feet on your desk.

TELE-MUSCLES

I wince whenever I see someone using a telephone headset. It's another example of being drawn into the "box." Reaching for the phone uses important shoulder, arm, and hand functions. Grasping the receiver is also useful work, as is holding it to your ear. For those whose work requires a headset, you should be doing the nonpain E-cise programs in chapter 6 as a way to replace the lost muscular demand.

I'm often asked if it is harmful to raise your shoulder to pin the receiver against your ear. There's no problem if your head and shoulders are in functional positions to start with. When you hang up the phone, they'll simply move back into proper alignment. The difficulty arises when the head (neck) and shoulder are misaligned by being rounded forward. If that's the case, you are reinforcing and strengthening the misalignment.

---

millions of years. Without our having to give it a thought, our more than six hundred skeletal muscles were regularly accessed, engaged, and put to work. Now modern men and women can do a day's labor using roughly two hundred muscles, or about 30 percent of the total. A few more are called on sporadically for walking and other activities. But the same "suspects" are rounded up day after day and made to toil away.

This is where the patterns come from and how they are reinforced. It's a variation on Parkinson's law: "Work expands to fit the time available." What's happening is that muscles and functions shrink to fit the work available. Obligingly, the work shrinks further, as technology evolves to replace muscles. There is a simultaneous and circular downsizing of muscles, work, and patterns of motion under way.

The noose is tightening. The PC "tiger cage" is actually spacious compared with the next step down. Modern life is increasingly conducted inside an invisible box floating directly in front of you that covers an area from about midthigh to the shoulders; and it's about the depth of a forearm, with the elbow bent at a ninety-degree angle.

Bingo! Our portable work zone. It makes the "tiger cage" look like a penthouse.

We bring work to this box, or it is carried to us by technology and tools. Move to the left or right, and the box travels along. All of us have heavy-duty, sophisticated musculoskeletal functions to handle chores within a much larger radius, but most people hardly ever use them. When they do—and immediately start feeling pain, discomfort, or restriction—they'll pull back inside the comfort zone of the box. Before long these vital functions are inaccessible.

Notice how rarely you reach outside of this box. When it happens, what do you feel? Is there stiffness? Do you have to work harder? More ominously, do you notice the creation of another even smaller box? A PC, particularly one with a keyboard that has a built-in pointing device, is creating a box within a box. Hand, wrist, arm, elbow, and shoulder movement all seem to be pulled down and into a seven-by-fifteen-inch area. The head is coming along for the ride, too. This wouldn't be a problem, however, if a fully functional musculoskeletal system were involved. In that case we'd be able to spend the day in almost any size box and climb right out again without strain.

Is it too late for that?

No. If you've been conscientiously doing your E-cise program, the body is raring to start breaking patterns.

Will it be easy?

Yes, surprisingly so. Start small with a few suggestions from the "Escapism" list earlier in this chapter, and build from there.

Picture Show

Patterns of motion carry over from work to play. It figures, really. The muscles and functions we rely on day after day are the ones that are readily accessible to support leisure and recreational activities. The problem is, we end up strengthening those "usual suspects" again.

Later in this chapter I'll provide you with an additional program of six E-cises to help break out of this pattern, but first I would like you to see how self-defeating it can be to "buff" your dysfunctions at a health club or on home gym equipment or just by going for a healthful walk around the block.

In figure 11.1, the model is working out on a treadmill, a favorite piece of equipment because it allows the gym rat to sweat without using

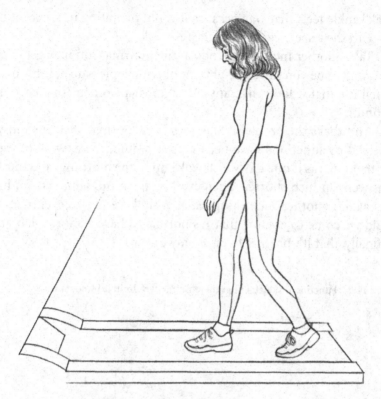

Figure 11.1 A treadmill workout that is not working out.

any of the right muscles. Like most people who sit down to work, her back is in flexion. Notice the lack of curve in the lower back, and the way her head and shoulders are rolled forward. By imagining a vertical line arising from her hip, you can see how out of position the head really is. This is helping to keep her hips rolled back, with the result that the muscles in the front and rear of the thighs are not engaged. There's stress in the hip's ball-and-socket joint and in the knees. She's waddling with her peripheral hip muscles rather than walking in a DROM gait pattern.

This woman likes the treadmill because she doesn't want to put a lot of impact on her right ankle, which is "weak," and the machine gives her a good aerobic blast. Actually, as she bypasses the prime movers in her thighs and hips, most of the aerobic benefits are lost. She's aerobically tuning her body to lesser, secondary muscles, which I believe destabilizes the cardiovascular system rather than strengthening it. The "weak" ankle feels that way because it is not operating in synchronization with the knee. And as a result it is weak.

Take another moment to look at the drawing. You may get it, and I certainly hope you do, but eight out of ten people who see this drawing tell me that it looks like any other normal woman (or man) on a treadmill.

And that's the problem! She does look "normal." Serious musculoskeletal dysfunctions have become so commonplace, we look right past them. It's as if one day we all woke up in the morning, and our left arms were an inch shorter. Then every year on the same date, it happens again: another inch disappears. Would we notice eventually, or would we come to assume that it's normal to have a shorter left arm? Or finally, that it's normal to have only one arm?

Figure 11.2   Functional skeletal alignment on the treadmill is important.

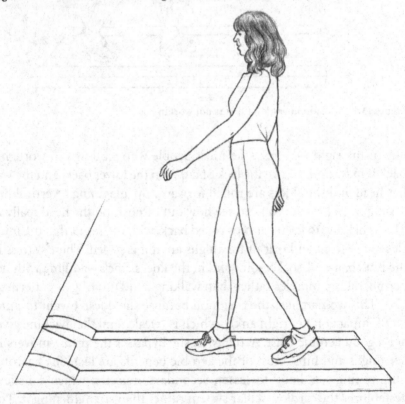

It's an extreme example, admittedly. Wouldn't we notice by comparing pictures of people from an earlier period? You'd think so, but there are plenty of pictures of people from fifty or a hundred years ago who did not walk or stand like our "normal" model. They also didn't have epidemics of RSI and chronic musculoskeletal pain that the Bureau of Labor Statistics reported cost $20 billion a year in workers' compensation claims.

In figure 11.2 the model is hitting the treadmill with her musculoskeletal system fully functional. Look at the head, shoulders, spine, and hips. The work is going to the right posture muscles. The joints are opening and closing smoothly.

When you are on a treadmill, which model do you resemble? The answer is an important one because it helps explain why your workout programs may not be working—or working *against* your fitness and health.

Bypassing prime movers to build strength in secondary muscles is the way to strengthen dysfunctions. Take a look in the gym's mirrors. Check your back and shoulders.

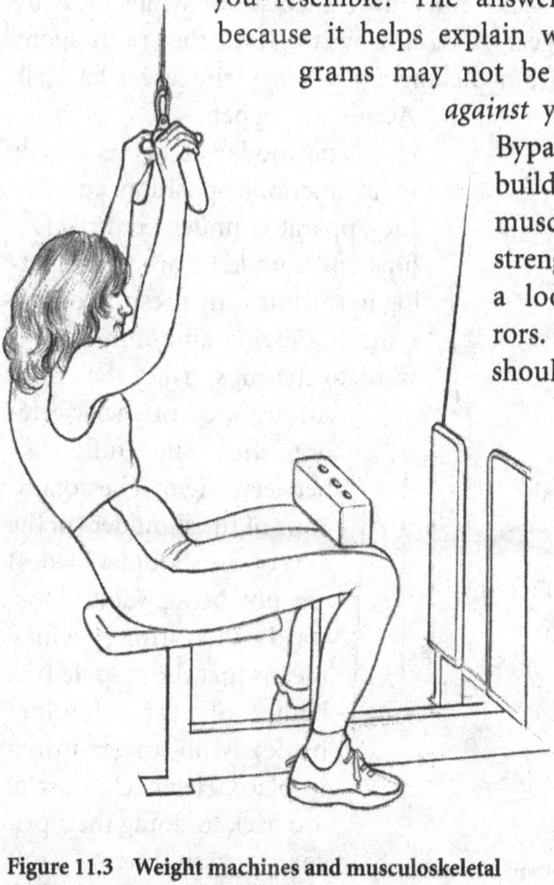

The model in figure 11.3 is using a popular overhead weight machine. She should stop what she's doing. As she pulls down on the bar, the curve in her spine is being flexed as though Robin Hood were drawing back the string on his trusty longbow. The vertebral disks of the spine

Figure 11.3 Weight machines and musculoskeletal dysfunctions are a bad combination.

are being squeezed under enormous pressure. To make matters worse, her right hip is actually engaging properly—the right foot indicates that by being pointed straight ahead—so the pressure on the spine isn't balanced left to right. Now it's like pinching the disk with a pair of pliers, using the force of whatever weight the machine is set on. Look at the head and shoulders—she is actually using her neck muscles to help bear the weight. It's going to do wonders for her headaches.

Personally, I love to lift weights. But this kind of stuff—and I'm showing you another "normal" view of what goes on in the weight room—drives me crazy. The equipment makers and health club owners avoid being bankrupted by liability suits only because their customers don't hurt themselves while they are using the gear. A month or two later, they're in agony from picking up a heavy suitcase. Oh, well. Accidents happen.

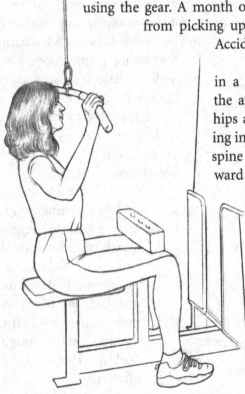

The model in figure 11.4 is in a functional position and has the apparatus under control. Her hips and shoulders are participating in the lifts. Any pressure on the spine is flowing smoothly downward to the hips, using the entire surface area of each vertebra and the full disk between them. The rotator cuffs of the shoulder (in the area of the shoulder blades) are not being yanked forward this time, which means that the scapula (the blade of the shoulder blade) is no longer frozen in place. Her neck muscles are back to doing their primary assignment—supporting the head.

Figure 11.4 Weight machines will not unduly stress properly aligned joints.

Figure 11.5 Hip and back flexion are detriments on stationary bikes.

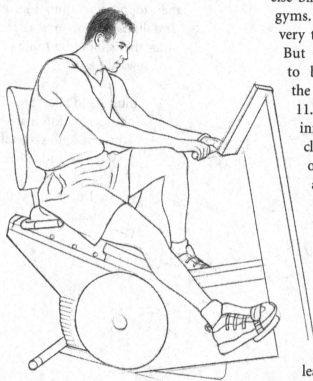

Like treadmills, exercise bikes are popular in gyms. "Spinning" is very trendy these days. But you don't want to be spinning like the model in figure 11.5. He is giving his inner-thigh muscles a great workout. These muscles are strong anyway, since he uses them for walking and holding himself in chairs. But the more powerful they become, the more difficult it is to release the hips from flexion. That's why his back is shaped like a C. He is leaning slightly to the left to get his thoracic back muscle—about midway up—to kick in and help the inner thigh muscles. This creates a situation where the bike rider is conditioning his back muscles to help him walk. In time he will wonder why his midback is so stiff and sore. Must be his PC.

In figure 11.6 the model's thoracic back muscles are minding their own business—supporting the thoracic back. The muscles in the front of his thighs—the quadriceps—are engaged, as are the glutes and hamstrings, located on the backs of the thighs and buttocks. This stabilizes the knees and ankles.

The same thing is happening outside the gym. Bikers, runners, in-line skaters, and weekend athletes of all sorts aren't getting the full benefits of the time and money they are investing in physical fitness. Tragically, many of them are actually undermining their health. Poised

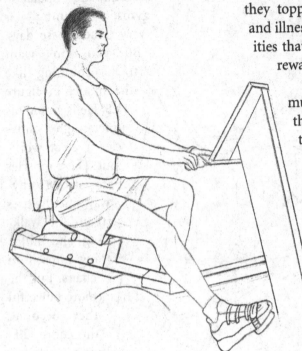

Figure 11.6　A stationary bike delivers full benefits to a functional rider.

on the edge of injury by their lifestyles and occupations, they topple over into injury and illness by pursuing activities that should be fun and rewarding.

Our priorities must be to take care of the foundation first— the musculoskeletal system—and then rebuild strength, health, and well-being.

Restoring the Foundation

Occasional, moderate, and power PC users may just add the E-cise menu in this section as a prelude or warm-up to their regular exercise and recreational routines. If you are still feeling pain or stiffness after a couple of weeks of doing your daily E-cise program for pain, double-check to make sure you are following the instructions. Also, slow down. Sometimes we're in a rush to get through them, and it impairs the performance. By all means put your other conditioning and training activities on hold—no running, weights, and the like. Playing through the pain is a loser's game.

When you are pain free, use these next six E-cises as a prelude to your favorite workout or as a stand alone program once or twice a week, if you're in the mood for extra activity.

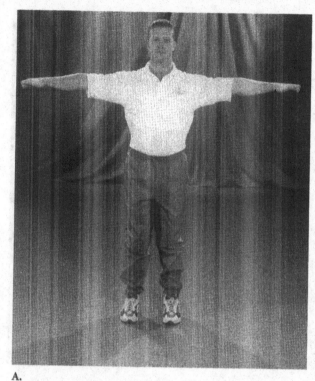

A.

This E-cise gives the shoulders a chance to use their ball-and-socket joints. Shoulder joints hinge forward and back and rotate in a ball-and-socket configuration. When we pitch a softball it's the shoulder's ball-and-socket doing the work. Likewise, serving a tennis ball relies on the ball-and-socket. But rowing a boat with a pair of oars takes the shoulder's hinge function (paddling a canoe uses both). Operating a mouse or keyboard means a lot of forward hinge demand, which often locks the shoulders in that forward position. It can happen in either the right or left shoulders—or both at the same time. Arm Circles counteract that tendency.

Stand with your head up, feet parallel about a hip-width apart, and arms at your sides. Curl the fingers of each hand into a light fist with your thumbs straight. (This is known as a "golfer's grip.") Raise your arms out to your sides, until they are level with your shoulders. If one shoulder wants to pop up or swing forward, lower both until they stay level. (Pay attention to this, too, when you start doing the circles.) Keep the elbows and arms straight, palms down, and your thumbs pointing forward (a). Lift your arms. Now squeeze your shoulder blades together slightly, and rotate the arms forward in the direction the thumbs are pointing. Make a roughly six-inch-diameter circle. Keep your wrists and elbows straight—the circles must come from the shoulders. Do this twenty-five times at a slow to moderate pace. Reverse the circles by turning the palms up and thumbs back (b). Crank the thumbs around so that your palms are level. Do another twenty-five. Then repeat back the

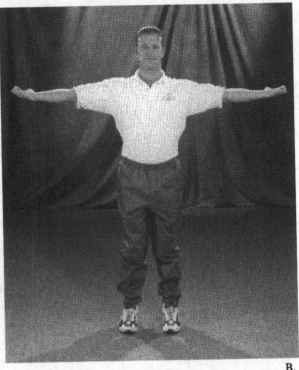

B.

other way for another twenty-five, and repeat again with the same count to the rear, so that you do a total of fifty in each direction. Remember to breathe.

• ELBOW CURLS

Now it's the hinges' turn. This E-cise activates the shoulders' hinge function. It also protracts and retracts the shoulder blades across the rib cage to prevent them from getting stuck in the forward position. If you like to swim, this will give you more power with overhand strokes and help the backstroke. It also aids balance when you're back on dry land walking, running, biking, or in-line skating.

Stand with your feet parallel, a hip-width apart. With your hands in the golfer's grip (see Arm Circles), place the flat area on the back of the index and middle fingers, between the first and second knuckle joints, on the temples in front of your ears; the thumbs extend downward, parallel with the cheeks. Draw your elbows back evenly and in line with the shoulders (a). Don't allow one shoulder to be lazy and not come all the way back. From this starting position, slowly swing your elbows forward until they touch in front (b). Keep your knuckles touching your temples, the thumbs fully extended. Your head should stay erect, not wobble or seesaw. Equalize the work and tension in both sides. Breathe deeply. Do twenty-five Elbow Curls. Each time your elbows touch counts as one curl. If you can't do twenty-five at first, reduce the number and slowly build up to it.

A.

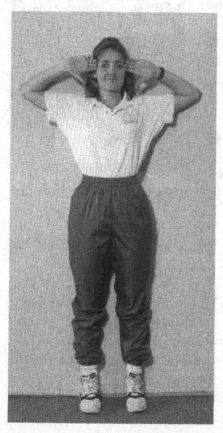

B.

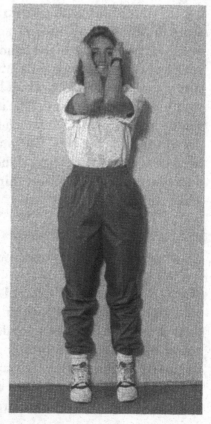

● STANDING OVERHEAD EXTENSION

This E-cise provides three important
services: It opens up the thoracic back
and the abdominal cavity, it increases
oxygen flow, and it strengthens the
muscles of extension in the back. It's a
big help to weight lifters, ballet
dancers, and even chess players.

Stand with your feet parallel, a
hip-width apart. Draw your head and
shoulders back, and roll your hips
forward into extension. You want an
arch in your lower back. Interlace the
fingers of your hands with the palms
toward your stomach. Raise your
arms, fingers still entwined, straight
over your head, and roll the palms of
your hands toward the ceiling. Make
sure your shoulders are back and
your hips still in extension. The arms
should be on either side of the head,
lightly touching the ears. Tip your
head back and look upward at the
back of your hands. Hold for thirty seconds. Remember to breathe,
which will be difficult at first.

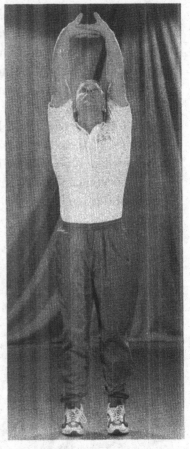

● STANDING SPREAD FOOT FORWARD BEND

This E-cise (figures 11.7a, b, and c) is one of my bulldozers. It puts
your hips into a neutral position and allows your prime movers to
do their jobs without the secondary muscles getting in the way. If
you're a golfer, you'll add power to your tee shots just because of the
improved weight transfer in your hips.

Stand with your legs spread about three to three and a half feet
apart. Keep your feet pointed straight ahead and flat on the floor.

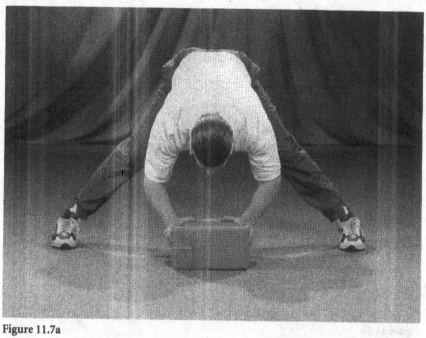

Figure 11.7a

Figure 11.7b

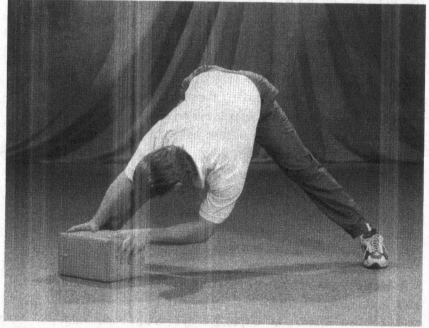

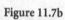

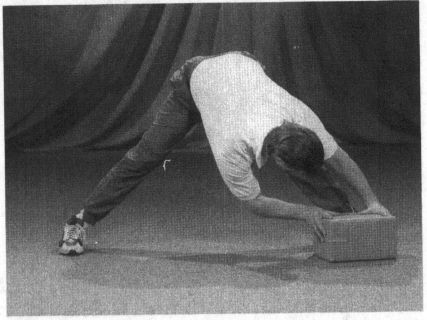

Figure 11.7c

(Don't let them roll.) Bend over at your hips and touch the floor directly in front of you. If that's too difficult, you may use a block, book, or other prop for support to rest your hands on. Tighten your thighs, and relax your torso toward the floor (a). Hold this position for one minute. Next, without straightening up again, slide your hands to your right foot (moving the prop, if you're using one). Keep both thighs tight and your torso relaxed (b). Hold that position for one minute. Then, slide left to the center briefly before moving your hands to your left foot (c). Again, keep your thighs tight and torso loose. Hold for one minute. Finally, move to the center, bend your knees, and roll your torso upright from the hips.

• STATIC EXTENSION POSITION

This E-cise is a powerful muscle relaxant. It releases the contracted muscles in your trunk and builds strength in your hips. You'll find this a big help if you play "explosive" sports like basketball,

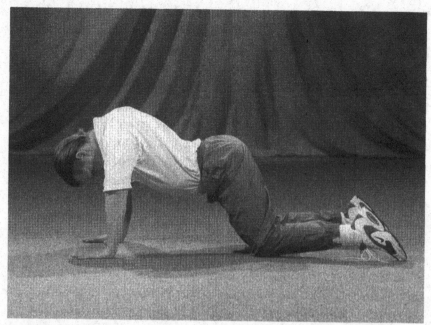

volleyball, and tennis. In general, though, there isn't a sport or activity that doesn't benefit from relaxed trunk muscles and stronger hips.

Get down on the floor on your hands and knees. Your hands should be about six inches forward of your shoulders to start, rather than directly under them. Let your back and head relax toward the floor as the shoulder blades come together. Relax. There should be a pronounced arch in your back. Keep your arms straight, and shift your hips forward six to eight inches so that they are not aligned with the knees. This will also bring your shoulders into line over your wrists. Hold for one to two minutes.

• CATS AND DOGS

If you have trouble understanding the principle of flexion and extension, this E-cise will at least let you feel it. As the cat flexes and the dog extends, this E-cise strengthens muscles and functions in a coordinated sequence. You need to break out of flexion to maximize the benefits of any sport, gym routine, or physical activity. This

E-cise provides total range of motion in the pelvis and the back in an anatomically correct and safe manner. It promotes breathing and better circulation. It's very effective, as you may know if you've done yoga.

Get down on the floor on your hands and knees. Make a "table" by aligning your hands under your shoulders and your knees and thighs under your hips. Your arms should be straight and your thighs parallel to them. Keep your legs and feet parallel to each other, as well. The feet are relaxed and resting across the top side of the toes, not flexed or up on the toes. Make sure your weight is distributed evenly. Smoothly round your back upward as your head curls under, to create a curve that runs from the buttocks to the neck—this is a cat with an arched back (a). Smoothly sway the back down while bringing your head up—this is the perky dog (b). Make these two moves continuously back and forth—don't keep them choppy and distinct. Do one set of ten. Exhale as you move into the cat position, inhale during the dog. Make sure, with the dog, that

A.

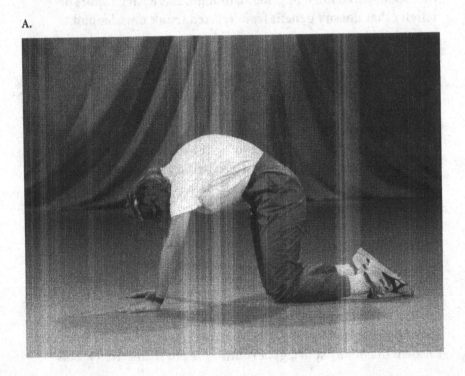

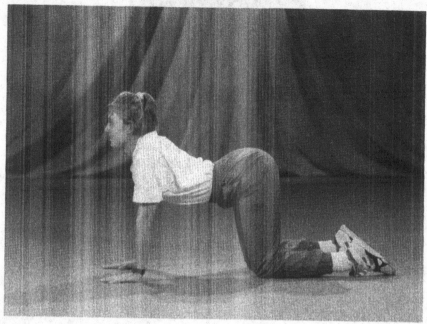

B.

your head comes fully back and up so that you are looking straight ahead and your shoulder blades collapse toward each other. Take your time. The pace should be slow, but not so slow that it breaks the flow between the cat and dog positions.

Does all this seem like more than you bargained for? If it does, try the programs for a week. Then evaluate where you stand. Ask yourself, "Is there still pain?" "Has it diminished?" "Has it moved?" "How do I feel overall?" Don't be too quick to decide. Many of us expect to be disappointed and jump to the conclusion that therapy isn't working when, in fact, we've made great progress. For instance, if the pain was constant before the E-cise program started and becomes intermittent after a week, you're gaining ground. Don't stop now!

Remember, even if you are in your twenties or thirties (or a teenager, unfortunately), these dysfunctions have been digging in for years. They won't disappear instantly. And they will never let go until you take responsibility for your own health.

12

JUST THE FAQS

"The worst downside of carpal tunnel surgery is that it is unnecessary and will ultimately fail."

I spend most of my workday answering questions, even though I've found that the best answer, quite often, is another question. This Socratic dialogue is a way to learn about our health and our responsibilities for maintaining it. The human body is my favorite teacher.

I've assembled here some questions that we frequently field at the clinic:

Q: If the PC at work isn't causing wrist pain, why does my wrist stop hurting over the weekend when I'm at home and resume first thing Monday morning as I boot up? It seems like cause and effect to me.
A: The reason the pain goes away over the weekend is that you've changed the demand on your body. In other words, the motion requirements at home are different from those at work. If you spend all day Saturday in the car doing errands or Sunday afternoon in front of the TV watching football, your muscles and joints aren't being stimulated in the same way. Even if a more strenuous routine is involved—gardening, home improvement, a pickup basketball game—there may be enough function or dysfunctional compensation to avoid overt pain symptoms over the short run. These functions that are being put to use

relatively briefly on the weekend are not the same ones being utilized for forty hours a week on the job. Give them time, and they too will start to hurt.

Take a fairly basic example. A serious runner—and carpal tunnel syndrome sufferer—will clock several miles of road work on her day off and feel great. She's not using her wrists and hands—therefore, she feels no pain. It seems like a great weekend, but she doesn't notice that her knees are gradually getting tender and unstable. It may take months of weekend running before she is aware that there is a problem—a problem that is coming from the same source as her sore wrists and hands: weak posture muscles and skeletal misalignment.

Meantime, she goes back to work Monday morning and doesn't put much demand on her knees and ankles. It's her arms, wrists, and hands that are taking a beating. In both cases the stress is coming from the musculoskeletal dysfunction. Now she's feeling one and not the other. Eventually, both will be heard from.

Q: Can I take painkillers and still do the E-cises?

A: You certainly can, but keep in mind that the drugs will mask the pain and interfere with *you* making an accurate assessment of the effectiveness of the E-cises. Pain is a message. If you pay attention to that message—where it's coming from, its intensity, and its other qualities—you'll know how your body is responding to treatment. One of my cardinal rules is: If it hurts, stop doing it. But if you're taking a painkiller, you won't know if it hurts. In that case who's in charge? Who makes the decision to go on or to stop?

This question really addresses the need to take a more direct and active role in managing one's health. If your PC suddenly started making strange sounds or the screen display changed colors, you'd be wide awake. But many of us are oblivious to the same kind of messages sent by the body. If we do a better job of tuning in, we can develop a very accurate assessment of what the body needs. Then we can make the decision rather than being passive.

One of the strengths of the Egoscue Method is that it is self-reinforcing. The E-cises go right to work: Positive changes occur, you know you're gaining on the problem, and so you keep at it. The validation is almost immediate. When you take painkillers, that payoff isn't as pronounced. There could be a tendency to slack off the therapy. In that way the drug is acting as a disincentive.

One other factor is that the E-cises will change your metabolic rate, since they engage the major posture muscles. As a result, a smaller dosage may be needed and that's on top of the pain alleviation that is already occurring from the E-cise. You could end up overmedicating yourself.

Notice that I'm not providing a yes or no answer. I'm giving you information so that *you* can reach a yes or no decision.

Q: Did I aggravate my carpal tunnel problem by playing the guitar? Would it be better to choose hobbies that don't require so much finger and wrist involvement?
A: No, and no. The PC's keyboard didn't cause the pain, nor did the guitar's strings. By going after the underlying musculoskeletal problems, you can do both without pain. Plucking or strumming the strings and playing the chords on a guitar are quite different from operating a PC keyboard. To play the instrument, the musician brings a different demand to the body, which is very desirable. The more stimulus and the more varieties of stimulus, the better! You'd lose that by giving up the guitar, and you'd lose access to the functions involved.

Furthermore, I believe that our choice of hobbies is an accurate gauge of what gives us pleasure. Work may not be enjoyable, but we do it anyway for the paycheck. The urge to play the guitar confirms that you know instinctively that the instrument is not causing the pain. You wouldn't give the guitar a second thought if it were really hurting you. We need to relearn the ability to listen to what the body is telling us.

Q: If alignment is so important, why does the body allow the skeleton to fall into misalignment?
A: The body doesn't discriminate between good and bad stimuli. It's all the same. What the environment hands out, the muscles, joints, and other components absorb. This anything-and-everything-goes approach assumes that the environment in due course will ask us to walk, run, stretch, leap, bend at the waist, make throwing motions, pull, push, carry heavy burdens, twist, turn, crawl, squat, and so on. Every

function was engineered by environmental demand that came at us from every direction. It's the secret of our survival skills as a species. The ultimate opportunists, we respond to our surroundings.

As the ultimate inventors and problem-solvers, we changed our surroundings as well. What's happening with skeletal misalignment is that the environment has stopped offering the rich, wide range of motion demand that it did in the past. But as always, the body is taking the available stimuli and using them. Only now the stimuli are no longer balanced. They come at us in limited, specific forms. Meanwhile, the parts that aren't being stimulated weaken and are soon overpowered by those that are getting more use. Unfortunately, it's mostly the peripheral and secondary muscles that are prospering at the expense of the prime movers and big posture muscles. Without these "heavy hitters," skeletal alignment is compromised. Once that happens, the body has no built-in mechanism to restore equilibrium—other than motion. It's a real catch-22.

Unlike our ancestors, we have the power and technology to shape our own environment in large and small ways. Until we deliberately replace this lost motion, the musculoskeletal system is in trouble and our health is in jeopardy.

Q: Fifteen years ago I used to spend several hours a day using a typewriter without any problem. I had to change jobs this year because the PC was killing me. Isn't there a difference in the keyboards that accounts for this?
A: It would be a cinch to rig up an old Remington manual typewriter to function as a PC keyboard. To input data, you'd be required to insert a sheet of paper, roll it through, and align the margins. Then you'd hammer away at the keys, banging on the "shift," and stopping at the end of each line to flick the lever to get the carriage to return to start another line. When you made a mistake, you'd have to pump the "backspace" key several times, erase, and retype. What a great workout!

The problem is, the "information highway" would run right off a cliff. A keyboard requiring that kind of demand would make Ralph Nader's old Corvair seem as safe and benign as a Volvo. There'd be lawsuits, congressional hearings, and federal regulations to curb the epidemic of pain caused by . . . ? That's right, the Remington manual typewriter.

Most of us no longer have the posture muscles required to sit in front of a typewriter for several hours, the way Great-Aunt Gladys did. If you went back to a typewriter and tried to do a PC's work with it, you would be in worse pain than you are right now. In the intervening fifteen years, the level of the "motion ocean" that kept you afloat has receded dramatically. Those musculoskeletal functions are high, dry, and largely inaccessible. The increasing incidental rate of chronic pain associated with the PC indicates that the level is still dropping.

Q: You don't seem to stress monitor or keyboard placement. Why is that?
A: Fiddling with the monitor and keyboard is a form of symptom management. It does not address the source of the problem or prevent it from happening in the first place.

I've watched many PC users at work in front of video monitors that have been adjusted to account for the chair, the workstation, and the individual's height. "Set the monitor at eye level," the mantra goes. Within a matter of minutes, this careful arrangement is made irrelevant by the head moving forward and down toward the screen. I half expect to hear a giant sucking sound and see them disappear into the monitor. As for the keyboard, moving it higher or lower will change the body's response to the task in superficial ways, but the basic misalignment problem is still there, still creating friction and stress. No matter what you do with the keyboard, rounded shoulders and a slumping back will always prevail.

To see what I mean, put both your hands on a PC keyboard in the typing position. Pull your head and shoulders all the way back while watching your hands. Notice that the wrist end of the hand is being raised via the action of the elbow. Now let the shoulders and back relax; the wrist and hand are being pushed down by the elbow. Move the keyboard lower, and this will still happen. Plus, the back rounds more. Raise it, change the angle, and the elbows gain even more of a mechanical advantage against the wrist.

If you're experiencing chronic pain, you may have discovered that its intensity varies according to the way you address the keyboard. You get "comfortable" by sitting on your right side and hunching the left shoulder, or fall into some other contortion. All that means is that the friction is being transferred to another less sensitive location. After a while, it will start to hurt there, too.

Q: I wasn't having any problem with my PC until I lost about twenty-five pounds. Can you explain that?
A: The chances are good that your weight-loss routine burned off muscle along with fat, leaving the body with even less capacity to maintain an upright posture. Don't forget that the reason fat is so hard to get rid of is that the body is programmed to store excess calories in case there's a famine. This surplus is a valuable commodity in an environment of scarcity. We actually protect it by first burning muscle tissue for energy once the intake of calories drops below a subsistence level. The body only reluctantly draws down its store of fat.

We really are superb managers of resources. From a musculoskeletal standpoint, the body has a way of making fine adjustments to avoid a crisis. We can live for months or years on the edge of chronic pain without being aware that anything is wrong. Suddenly, an event comes along to tip the balance—like muscle loss from a crash diet—and there's pain.

By the way, don't even think about fixing the problem by regaining the twenty-five pounds! You need to work on building muscle and activating functions with the E-cises in chapters 6 through 9.

Q: Is there an ideal sport or recreational activity that will help me avoid chronic pain?
A: All of them. With the possible exception of bungee jumping, popular mainstream sports and recreational activities are ideal chronic pain antidotes because they provide motion that would otherwise be unavailable. Bear in mind, though, that since most of us work more than we play, the dysfunctions we feed on the job are brought home on the weekend.

The guy who rarely so much as turns a doorknob on Monday to Friday goes to a tennis court on Saturday, where he performs the exact same functional motion to deliver a wicked forehand across the net. He hits the ball dozens of times—hard! When his elbow starts hurting, he concludes that tennis is to blame and gives it up. And that's too bad. He loses out on the benefits of the motion without curing the tennis elbow, which will become PC elbow or calculator elbow or cash register elbow.

The chronic pain is not caused by the sport or the demands of a job. The back, shoulder, and upper arm are designed to work with the elbow to pronate and supinate the hand (move the palm to face up or down). But our friend has rounded shoulders, which can't rotate. It means the elbows do most of the work. Eventually, there's a breakdown. Whereupon we hear the five words I dread the most: "I got hurt playing ————." Followed by the next five: "So I gave it up."

I recommend that you make an effort to vary your sports and recreational activities. We often end up playing with the muscles we work with because they are strong in the first place. One of the reasons for the biking boom is that it is an ideal sport for someone who sits in a chair all day and whose hips and back are locked in flexion.

Q: Is there a sport to avoid, like running?
A: No, no, no. We were designed to run. People get hurt running, or while performing any sport, primarily because they are attempting to run or play with weakened and unstable musculoskeletal systems. Most sports accidents—football included—could be avoided if the players came to the game with fully functional bodies.

Q: I'm considering carpal tunnel surgery. It sounds fairly straightforward. What's the downside?
A: I don't know, and neither does your doctor. There isn't enough reliable research on what really happens over the long run to a wrist whose transverse carpal ligament has been surgically severed. I'll give you my opinion, though. The ligament is in there for two reasons: strength and stability. For me, those are convincing reasons for leaving it alone. Ask your physician questions like "Will I recover full hand and wrist function?" and "How do you define full hand and wrist function?"

The answer to this second question can be very revealing. Often you'll be told that the hand will probably be *close* to normal, but you won't be able to "do handstands" or work as many hours as you once did on the PC. To me, that's *not* normal.

The worst downside of carpal tunnel surgery is that it is unnecessary and will ultimately fail. The problem is lack of function and misalignment. That's not going to be cured by surgery.

Q: I've seen exercises for carpal tunnel syndrome that work directly on the hand and wrist, such as balling your hand into a fist and releasing, or straightening the wrist and relaxing the fingers. Why is your E-cise approach so different?

A: Sorry about answering a question with another question. But what happened the last time you got a kick in the shins or caught your fingers in the door? You rubbed the injury, and it felt better because more blood and oxygen were being sent to the area. Therapy that works directly on a painful wrist, elbow, neck, or shoulder is doing the same thing. Most of the chronic pain we are discussing in this book comes from either nerve impingement or inflammation. Both types involve restricted oxygen flow. Direct therapy addresses that but doesn't affect the underlying problem.

Q: Won't wrist and back braces solve the problem of skeletal misalignment?

A: They merely shift the problem elsewhere. Worse, braces usurp functions that need to be strengthened, not isolated and immobilized. A third reason to avoid braces is that they interfere with the close interactions of the body's various structural components. If you change how the elbow or wrist operates, it affects the shoulder and the neck. Once that happens, every part of the body is in play.

But I'm glad the question arose, because there will be more on this subject in the next chapter.

Q: Can I do the E-cises after surgery?

A: If you mean "Is it too late after surgery to do the E-cises?" the answer is no, it's never too late to restore lost musculoskeletal functions. Alignment is not going to happen by itself—at least not for most modern men and women. The E-cises are the best vehicle for achieving that objective before or after surgery.

Q: From what you say about alignment, it seems like good posture is the key to avoiding pain. Wouldn't it be enough to pay attention to sitting up straight and keeping your head and shoulders back?

A: It can't be done. As soon as we shift our focus off the command—"Sit up straight"—and start doing something else, our posture goes back to autopilot and our dysfunctions take over. By strengthening muscles and accessing the proper functions, we are reprogramming the autopilot to keep us in alignment without having to think about it.

Q: I don't have pain, and I don't want pain. But how will I know when I can safely stop doing the E-cises?
A: Read my lips—N-E-V-E-R. I'm afraid that our "motion ocean" is going to keep on receding. Just as we have to feed ourselves, we must dish up a daily minimum requirement of motion. It's a life sentence, but the good news is that the more you move, the more you want to move. Movement is a chore only when we're dysfunctional. In that case the pleasure is gone.

Watch young children. They move for the sheer joy of it. Adults think we outgrow this exuberance. What's happening, though, is that we grow into a culture that expects proper adults to be "still." It is stillness, not aging, that deprives us of our instinctive love of motion.

Q: I still don't get flexion and extension, particularly when it comes to the hips.
A: Join the crowd. Think of the pelvis as forming a big hinge where it joins with the spine. Bend over and touch your toes—the hinge closes (full flexion). Stand straight—the hinge opens (full extension). The problem is that when most people stand up, they are not straight—they are still in partial flexion; the hinge never opens completely. I can demonstrate this if you'll sit on the floor, squarely on your bottom, with your feet straight out in front. Without using your hands on the floor for support, square your shoulders and straighten your back. Okay, now put an arch in your lower back. No hands! No seesawing back and forth. It's tough. Most people can't do this because I'm asking them to fully open the hip-hinge. Key muscles of the pelvis aren't strong enough to obey. One of the reasons is that the contracting muscles that hold the hinge closed in partial flexion get so much use, they are stronger than those that open the hinge. By asking you to sit on the floor to arch your back, I'm making you rely almost exclusively on these weak pelvis muscles to achieve extension, rather than helping out with knee, thigh, and thoracic back contortions. If you repeat the demo standing up, and pay close attention to your knees, you find that they

are tightening appreciably when you try to arch your back. The knee-hinge is opening fully and attempting to go past full extension (by twisting or popping) to compensate for the partial opening of the hip-hinge. The knee is attempting to flip the hip back into the proper extended position. It's another example of how one dysfunctional component puts stress on another. In this case, the lazy hips are getting a free ride at the expense of the hard-working knees. Eventually, the knees will start breaking down. We need to get all the body's hinges to open and close without restriction or extra stress by eliminating muscular imbalances.

In figure 12.1 the model is doing two things. He is thinking, and he has put himself into flexion. The pose is reminiscent of the famous sculpture *The Thinker* by Rodin. It's interesting that we associate this posture with introspection and intellectual activity. In contrast there is the monumental *David*, hewn out of marble by Michelangelo. The biblical giant-killer stands tall in full extension, ready to take action. We have to work to preserve both of these inherent musculoskeletal capabilities. Go ahead, think; lean forward and study the situation closely. Then get up and go do something about it. Flexion and extension; thought and action.

Q: **Women have more flexibility in their hips. Does that make them more vulnerable to chronic pain?**
A: No, the body is very democratic. Men and women are equally vulnerable to chronic pain if there is insufficient proper motion to maintain their musculoskeletal systems. Women need to watch out for socially mandated roles and expectations

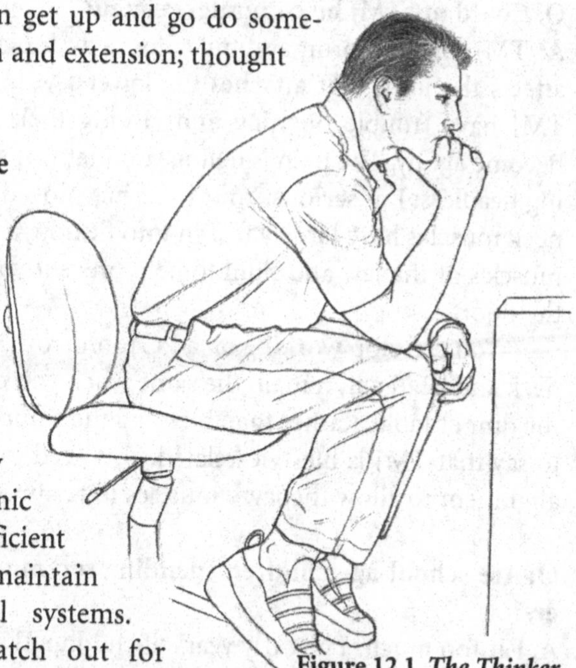

Figure 12.1 *The Thinker* goes digital.

that assign them to a more motionless status than men. It makes my day to see women in hard hats and getting paid to slam-dunk a basketball.

I know, however, that many women bristle at the idea that they are "motionless." Modern women are busy; they work hard. But distinctly unequal patterns of motion are commonplace. Women, for example, are not expected to have more than minimal upper body strength. Watch otherwise-fit and hugely competent female road warriors struggle to get luggage into the overhead storage compartment on an airplane. Often a male passenger will help out. It's assumed that he has the required upper-body strength (even though he may not).

I'm not knocking good manners. My point is that gender stereotyping leads us to accept the idea that lack of upper-body strength is okay in women. It's not. There are health consequences. Among them are headaches, stiff necks, lack of balance, and osteoporosis. The major posture muscles in the upper body are necessary to maintain skeletal integrity.

Q: Could my TMJ be computer related?

A: TMJ, or temporomandibular joint dysfunction, is a disorder that affects the joint that attaches the lower jaw to the skull. People with TMJ have trouble opening and closing their mouths. Chewing can become agony. The pain is telling you that you are in danger of becoming headless. I'm serious. Your head has moved so far forward that the neck muscles have largely frozen into flexion, and they've recruited the muscles of the jaw and skull to help prevent your head from falling to the floor.

You can stop working on a PC tomorrow, but the position of your neck and head will remain the same when you drive, watch TV, or sit at the dinner table. Rather than blaming the computer, it is more accurate to say that TMJ is lifestyle-related. You need to restore vertical skeletal alignment to allow the jaw's muscles to resume their proper functions.

Q: Are school-age children spending too much time using computers?

A: Far too much. The early years of childhood are extremely important for developing stable musculoskeletal structure and function. The only way that can happen is for kids to spend hours on the move. It's not necessary for them to be athletes or fitness freaks; if they get out into the world, they'll find trees to climb and puddles to jump.

Once the foundation is in place, young people can spend as much time as they want studying or playing games on a computer. But like adults, they'll have to feed themselves motion in large enough helpings to keep their functions from crumbling. It is particularly true if we continue to insist that children need to work more and play less. Recess and athletic programs are vanishing from many of our schools, replaced by academic activities that are designed to prepare students for top colleges and careers. Let's hear it for the fast track! But I doubt that people in chronic pain can be among the very best, brightest, and fastest for long.

Q: How much motion is enough?

A: I hate that question. It begs for a pat answer—"Twenty minutes a day is enough for every man, woman, and child." And that's nonsense. For some people twenty minutes is enough. Their environment is richer in motion, and it supplies the rest of what's needed. Others aren't so lucky. They may need an hour or more.

On the other hand, there's no such thing as too much motion when the body is functional. That doesn't mean you're Superman. At some point fatigue will set in, and the body will tell you in no uncertain terms to stop and rest. But I don't have much sympathy for the less-is-more school of fitness that is being advocated these days. I believe there is a direct positive correlation between the time we spend in active motion and the time we spend pain free.

13

DESPERATE MEASURES— MEASURES— SURGERY, DRUGS, AND ERGONOMICS— DON'T WORK

"Ergonomics practices serial sacrifice—serial carnage—as we destroy joint after joint, function after function, in the crusade for ergonomic solutions."

Gil is my poster boy. I've written about him before, and I'll probably keep telling his story because it perfectly captures the paradigm of pain.

Gil was on the move a lot and traveled light. He didn't lug around a notebook computer or personal digital organizer. The most important item in his carry-on luggage was a single fingerless glove, rumpled and well worn. It covered his right hand like a second skin, reminiscent of what gunslingers once wore.

I'm not sure, but I'd guess Gil was computer illiterate. He never bothered to turn on a PC or surf the web (although he'd probably like playing Doom). What he enjoyed was a sport that historians seem to think was invented in an eighteenth-century Irish jail.

He could play a mean game of handball.

Gil was a national champion. Was. When he came to my clinic a few years ago, he was a wreck of a thirtysomething athlete, who wanted only to play and win just one more major tournament. This is how I recall our consultation:

"What's the problem?" I asked.

"My elbow hurts."

"I know. I can tell by the way you're holding it," I said. Surprised by the comment, he tried to move his right shoulder back, but it was rounded so far forward that it was nearly impossible to budge.

Gil was very candid. He explained that over the years the elbow pain had gotten increasingly severe. To play, he had resorted to frequent cortisone shots administered directly to the elbow joint.

I nodded, taking note of his use of the word *frequent*. Cortisone and frequent don't mix.

"Now I'm here because I can't have any more shots," Gil said.

"Why not?"

He stood up. "Feel my elbow."

I used my thumb and index finger like calipers to gently assess the swelling. With hardly any pressure at all, my thumb slid up and into the elbow capsule, pushing the skin before it like slipping on a glove. The thumb went in as far as the first joint. This didn't seem to give Gil any more pain than he was already enduring, but it was a total shock to me.

If you've ever been walloped by an elbow in the ribs or head, you know what a blunt instrument it is: a tough, three-way joint chock full of bone condyles, cartilage, tendons, and ligaments. I knew at once that numbed by cortisone, Gil had played and played until his elbow turned to mush.

There's not much that exercise therapy can do for a joint that has ceased to exist. So Gil had doctor-shopped. He moved from physician to physician conning them into cortisone treatments by not revealing his full medical history. Finally, the consequences were impossible to hide; no ethical doctor would provide another injection. Cortisone is just too destructive in large doses.

Gil killed the pain—temporarily—by permanently killing his elbow.

I tell this story because painkilling has become a huge industry. But we need to think carefully before buying its products and services. It's time to question whether seemingly more benign versions of cortisone are being administered in the form of surgery, drugs, and ergonomically correct devices to millions of people, with equally destructive effects.

Will we wake up in twenty or thirty years to find another author telling much the same story? Instead of Gil and his horribly mangled elbow, will it be a tale of young people with sore wrists or stiff necks, who wanted only to work without pain to build good lives? Will it be a tragedy of artificial joints, pills and their side effects, braces, and lives of lost mobility?

My prevailing optimistic side hesitates to answer—it's skittish about being disappointed. But the trends are not good. An estimated 120 million Americans suffer from some type of chronic pain. Pain is the leading cause of worker absenteeism, with 50 million lost days a year and $3 billion in lost wages. One out of six American households has someone with severe chronic pain. As for treatment costs, I've seen figures ranging from $100 million a year for carpal tunnel surgery to $100 billion to cover RSI-related conditions affecting computer users. Migraines, back pain, and arthritis ring up an estimated $40 billion; on top of that, ergonomic reengineering, the business of designing "worker-friendly" tools, furniture, and work space, takes in approximately $3 billion a year.

The statistics are frightening from at least two standpoints. One, the sheer number of people in pain; and two, the profit potential that is driving the search for pain cures into areas that may lead to quick short-term solutions that bring on long-term damage.

Let's start with the human toll. If roughly 40 percent of the U.S. population is in pain, it's time to ask a basic question: What is going on?

The answer is also quantifiable. A 1996 study by the U.S. Surgeon General found that 60 percent of the adult population are not physically active on a regular basis, 25 percent are not active at all, and half the young people between the ages of 12 and 21 are also not vigorously active.

Like the nesting Russian dolls that split open to reveal other smaller dolls inside, these figures on physical inactivity are the outer shell that holds the core reason for such enormously high rates of chronic pain. An executive summary that accompanied the study identified the source of chronic pain by being both bureaucratically oblique and precise at the same time:

> Regular activity that is performed on most days of the week reduces the risk of developing or dying from some of the leading causes of illness and death in the United States. Regular physical activity improves health in the following ways:
> Reduces the risk of dying prematurely.
> Reduces the risk of dying from heart disease.
> Reduces the risk of dying from diabetes.
> Reduces the risk of developing high blood pressure.
> Helps reduce high blood pressure in people who already have high blood pressure.
> Reduces the risk of developing colon cancer.
> Reduces the feeling of depression and anxiety.
> Helps control weight.
> Helps build and maintain healthy bones, muscles, and joints.
> Helps older adults become stronger and better able to move without falling.
> Promotes psychological well-being.
> Given the numerous health benefits of physical activity, the hazards of inactivity are clear. Physical inactivity is a serious nationwide problem. Its scope poses a health challenge to reducing the national burden of unnecessary illness and death.[1]

I agree that "The hazards of inactivity are clear," and my professional experience corroborates the study's findings. But unfortunately the government's message is likely to be ignored by its target audience. People do what gives them pleasure, and they avoid what doesn't. It's the reason that 60 percent of the U.S. population are not regularly active: Physical activity is unpleasant.

---

1. *The Surgeon General's Report on Physical Activity and Health,* July 11, 1996; Department of Health and Human Services, Washington, DC.

We are not by nature or culture sedentary, but in the last fifty years a sit-down, drive-by, tune-in, and kick-back lifestyle has eclipsed an older, established norm that provided a richer variety of motion and physical activity that, without conscious effort, kept our grandparents fit enough to derive pleasure from the effort. As a rule, they did not fall below a certain level of functionality until late in life.

My grandfather was an example. When I was ten or eleven, he reluctantly gave up his big house in the country and moved into town. One day I asked him if he missed his house. He replied, "Yes, I'd like to have those stairs back." I was amazed and wondered why in the world he missed that set of steep stairs to the second floor. He lived now in a nice one-level place with my aunt. I suggested he go to the park where there was a staircase he could climb. "It's not the same," Grandpa said.

It wasn't the same. I know that now. Those stairs were part of his life. The daily routine of trudging up and down the stairs had been broken. He looked back on them with pleasure and fondness, yet he wasn't about to climb the park's stairs just for the exercise. It wasn't long before his health began to fail.

Actually, Grandpa was lucky because at least he had a memory that linked pleasure with physical activity. If he had been allowed to go back home, it might have provided enough incentive for him to recover the functions he had so quickly lost by living on one level. But most of the inactive young people cited in the surgeon general's report don't have that advantage. Their functions haven't been lost—they were never developed in the first place. It's awfully hard to convince a teenager that physical activity is worthwhile when it is not only extremely unpleasant but, in many cases, painful.

We've spent a lot of time in this book discussing chronic pain symptoms—both pain and nonpain. Our inactivity as a nation is symptomatic of dysfunction: We don't move because physical activity is unrewarding, uncomfortable, or unpleasant. It explains the extraordinary levels of inactivity *and* chronic pain. We no longer move enough to cross the threshold where the value to be gained compensates for the effort being made. The consequence is chronic pain and the long list of illnesses that the surgeon general enumerated.

The Usual Business of Business as Usual

Any market that encompasses 120 million people is an irresistible target for profit-making businesses. For years I've been questioning the wisdom of 85 to 90 percent of the elective orthopedic surgery that is performed in the United States. We've been too quick to cut and be cut, mainly because there is an abundant supply of surgical talent and technology on hand. American doctors conduct surgery for lower back conditions five times more frequently than their British counterparts. Is that due to our genetically weaker backs? I doubt it. The more likely explanation is that the perennially cash-strapped British National Health Service opts for more economical and conservative treatment. The overwhelming majority of British physicians are GPs, not surgeons or other specialists. This is fortunate for the average Briton, since recent studies have shown that of the four possible courses of action—doing nothing, drug treatment, physical therapy, and surgery—surgery tends to be the least successful. (Doing nothing is the most successful, which I'll address below.)

Fortunately, the medical community has begun to recognize the problem. Increasingly, it is offering surgery as a last-resort option for many musculoskeletal problems, and patients are being strongly advised to consider less invasive procedures. Managed health care, in addition, has moved the United States somewhat closer to the British model, with the difference that private insurance companies, rather than the central government, are guarding the purse strings.

The downside is that drugs and gadgetry are assuming a larger role. They are cheaper than surgery, but both share the same defect: They treat a symptom, not the problem. Statistically, "doing nothing" is the most effective treatment for back pain because the patient actually does *something*. Motivated by the pain, he modifies his behavior (as does she). It doesn't take all that much. The body is so resilient and adaptable that simply resting for a few days or getting a new chair can be enough to alleviate musculoskeletal pain and keep it at bay for weeks or months. Of course, the underlying problem remains, even though the symptom abates temporarily.

A painkilling drug takes this a step farther into dangerous territory. It allows us to continue our behavior—no rest, no new chair—but it eliminates the pain symptom. Remember Gil? That's what cortisone did for him. He continued to play and continued to obliterate his elbow. The cortisone was destructive in its own way, but the mechanical abuse of the joint was equally to blame. Masking pain with anti-inflammatory drugs removes the incentive to take action that can give the body a fighting chance to respond to the problem in the short term. Business as usual means the usual business of traumatizing muscles and joints. As the damage accumulates, the drug's dosage must increase proportionally until pain finally breaks through or pops up in another place.

Many people who come to my clinic have been advised by their physicians that they have nerve damage. It's the equivalent of being told "there's nothing more we can do." But the diagnosis often turns out to be incorrect. The nerves have not been permanently damaged; they have merely been affected by skeletal misalignment and muscular dysfunction. Once those circumstances are corrected, the nerves return to health. I'm convinced that what we are seeing is the drug *mask* at work. The nerves are being rubbed, irritated, and impinged on beyond their level of tolerance, but the painkiller has pulled the plug on that circuit to prevent it from shutting down the system. In due course the nerves start showing signs of severe wear and tear.

Breathalyzers are now attached to automobile ignitions to prevent alcohol abusers from driving while intoxicated. I'd like to see something similar hooked up to a PC to stop those who are using painkillers from booting up. And that doesn't mean the PC is dangerous—the dysfunctional operator is dangerous to him or herself.

Something tells me Microsoft isn't about to add an *Egoscue-lyzer* to its Windows operating system, so I'll supply a warning right here on this screen:

> **GPF #1: If You've Taken a Painkiller for Musculoskeletal Pain**
> **Save Your Work**
> **Press Cancel**
> **Go Home**

I'm adamant about this, because relying on painkillers to go about business as usual is a huge mistake. The drug does nothing to eliminate the musculoskeletal problem that is causing the pain. That problem—let's assume for our purposes that it's a restricted elbow joint—is aggravated by arm movement. But you won't know that. The painkiller has numbed your elbow.

I can hear the excuse—and it's a good one: *I just need to finish this project.* Yet every time you reach for the mouse or tap the keys, you are damaging the elbow joint. We've got to stop making excuses—they're hurting us.

It is so easy and so misleading to fool ourselves into believing that when the pain goes away, the problem leaves with it. No. It happens only when we take action to strengthen muscles, restore skeletal alignment, and stabilize the entire musculoskeletal system.

Some prescription drugs and alcoholic beverages carry warnings about the hazards of operating automobiles and other potentially dangerous pieces of equipment while consuming those products. The warning label deserves to be plastered on your PC—not because the computer equipment is dangerous—it's being operated by a dysfunctional body that is a danger to your health.

The Workerless Workplace

Like drugs and surgery, ergonomic gadgets are also market-driven products and the product of good intentions. The whole idea is to help people. Even so, the massive reengineering of the workplace is actually a hindrance. For one thing, it persuades people that the problem has been solved and that no further effort on their part is required. This external solution to a set of internal circumstances breeds dependence on a never-ending series of technological "fixes." Gradually, we cede direct control of the world around us. But the subservience offers no payoff. Since it is only a temporary and symptomatic solution, the pain increases along with a sense of helplessness.

Second, it leads to a proliferation of symptoms and an escalating crisis. In almost every RSI case we see in the clinic, the individual presents multiple symptoms. Often they are the direct result of an ergonomic solution, like a new keyboard or a wrist brace, that shifted the problem from the wrist to the elbow, the shoulder, or the neck. The rationale is that the shift allows the injured or inflamed joint to heal. But that never happens because the source of the problem isn't addressed. The transfer becomes permanent, and as such it undermines another musculoskeletal component. Before long the pain spreads.

And the third strike against ergonomics is basic economics. The ultimate outcome of a worker-friendly, ergonomically correct workplace is a workerless place full of robots and automated systems. If we accept the idea that less motion is the desired end, the musculoskeletal system will grow weaker and less stable until any motion—no matter how limited—is excruciating. Perforce, business will replace humans with machines to lower costs and uncertainty, and to increase productivity. Even the simplest tasks, like pushing a button or turning a dial, require muscle power. If the ability to keep the body erect is compromised, even such trivial physical demands will overtax our resources. Jobs aren't going to just "go south," they are just going to go away.

Ironically, the logical fallacy to ergonomics is the belief that repetitive motion can be cured by repetitive motion. This fallacy rests on the assumption that there is good motion and bad motion. For instance, by raising the height of a work surface to eliminate the need to bend at the waist or crane the neck (bad), we are restricting the individual to mostly forearm and hand movement (good) for several hours a day. Meanwhile, key functions—bending forward, straightening up, stretching, and lateral movement—that support the spine and the ability to remain upright are not being utilized. They will weaken. In due course there will be back pain, but perhaps before that happens, the worker will enjoy a pleasant weekend at home in the garden with time for a little weeding. Suddenly, his or her back will go out. Is the ergonomic solution to blame? No, of course not. Weeding caused the problem!

The body's musculoskeletal functions are so balanced, unified, and interdependent that attempts to manage movement lead to innumerable unintended consequences. In the last example, no one set out to cause a back problem by changing the height of the work surface. Yet inevitably, such ergonomic tinkering attempts to improve upon the body's natural processes by choosing the right way to move (painless) as opposed to the wrong way (painful). Once the choice is made, the next step is to compartmentalize or isolate right from wrong. One compartment moves, the other doesn't.

That's where things turn ugly. As motion is restricted, supporting functions shared by the "good" and the "bad" are undermined or lost entirely. The quest to eliminate bad movement by administering concentrated doses of good movement actually leads to worse movement. This drags the ergonomic expert deeper into the role of redesigning the workers as well as the workplace. There are alternating episodes of *pain/pain abatement through motion management/and more pain* as ergonomics selects which functions are deemed necessary and discards those that are not. There's no stopping the merry-go-round. It wouldn't be a big deal if we were just talking about substituting one piece of furniture for another. This amounts to practicing surgery without a knife. The pile of discarded functions gets larger and larger.

Here's another example of motion management run amok, one that specifically applies to the PC. A wrist brace discards unrestricted flexion and extension in the wrist. The elbow is expected to replace the lost functions. But the normal rollover or crossover function of the two bones in the forearm is limited by the brace, which means that the elbow cannot perform this task very well and is under increased stress. The shoulder then gets involved, pulling the neck and upper back forward and down. Hence, the original dysfunction—loss of vertical alignment—is aggravated.

An ergonomically correct keyboard, mouse, workstation, or chair does basically the same thing. It shifts work to other musculoskeletal components. The dysfunctional muscular compensation that is already present responds with even more compensation. In the short run, there may be pain relief that convinces us that we are on the right track. But that's an illusion. All that is happening is that we are sacrificing another virgin to appease the gods of unintended consequences. A formerly functional elbow or other joint is now being thrown into a dysfunctional state. Misaligned and overtaxed, it too is headed for breakdown. Ergonomics practices serial sacrifice—serial carnage—as we destroy joint after joint, function after function, in the crusade to reengineer the human body.

Natural Acts

Earlier in the book, when we discussed design range of motion, I pointed out that the human body is capable of "doing what it can do." By that I mean that the ability to perform a given function—muscular contraction, joint articulation, or what have you—confirms that nothing unnatural is happening. A ballerina's ability to dance on her toes is natural; she has the supporting muscles and other mechanisms. But the ballerina cannot expect to use her body only for that one purpose. The body is a total unit. Its functions interact in a balanced way from head to foot. What the dancer does with her head is as important as what happens with her feet and toes.

A PC user is the functional antithesis of the ballerina: Work is done by ten fingers instead of ten toes. In both cases, though, being pain free depends on the total functional integrity of the body. If the ballerina wears a knee brace, she affects the interaction between the hip and the knee, and the hip, knee, and ankle. It will change the way she dances. Likewise, the PC user who wears a wrist brace is altering the interaction between the fingers and the wrist, and the fingers, wrist, elbow, and shoulder. Moreover, the kinetic chain doesn't stop there. For both of them, it extends down the back (and up) to the hips, knees, ankles, and feet.

At any point patching or reengineering a link in the chain will have a direct effect on all the others. The next major articulating joint down the line from the brace will get hit the hardest. Before long it too is a candidate for a brace, which makes vulnerable the next major articulating joint, and so on until the body is bundled and bandaged like an Egyptian mummy.

Preventive bracing or preventive ergonomic reengineering is just as bad. These musculoskeletal interrelationships are being changed no matter whether the worker is functional or dysfunctional. Insurance company rules that encourage companies to force workers to wear back braces are actually making pain and back problems more likely. The brace is designed to provide the back with a stronger foundation to allow for heavy lifting. But it prevents the hips—which are the strong foundation—from doing their job; they weaken as a result.

Many grocery store chains and trucking firms require that vestlike back braces be worn by their employees. Whenever I see a clerk or a driver wearing his or her brace undone, I ask about it. Every time they say, "Damned brace gets in my way!" And it does. Those are the functional workers speaking. They don't need the help. The dysfunctional workers do, but they end up losing what minimal hip strength and stability remains. When they go home without the brace, they are in maximum danger of injury because their hips have been reengineered right out of business.

I'll make a prediction: Before long some genius in an insurance company or the government is going to get the idea of requiring all PC users to wear wrist braces. They'll pass it off as being the same thing as forcing drivers and their passengers to wear seat belts. If and when that happens, we'll look back on 120 million people in chronic pain as the golden age of health and fitness.

My favorite illustration in this book, figure 13.1, is artist Wendy Wray's version of a Digital Age knight in a suit of armor. The original idea behind it was to show you the ridiculous position we're going to be in if we continue subscribing to the false promise of ergonomic solutions: *You've got mail!—But first put on your chain mail.*

What Wendy discovered, when she did her research, was that old suits of armor that are on display in museums all over the world are actually fossil records of the oldest and best brace of them all—the human body. The makers of suits of armor molded the product to fit

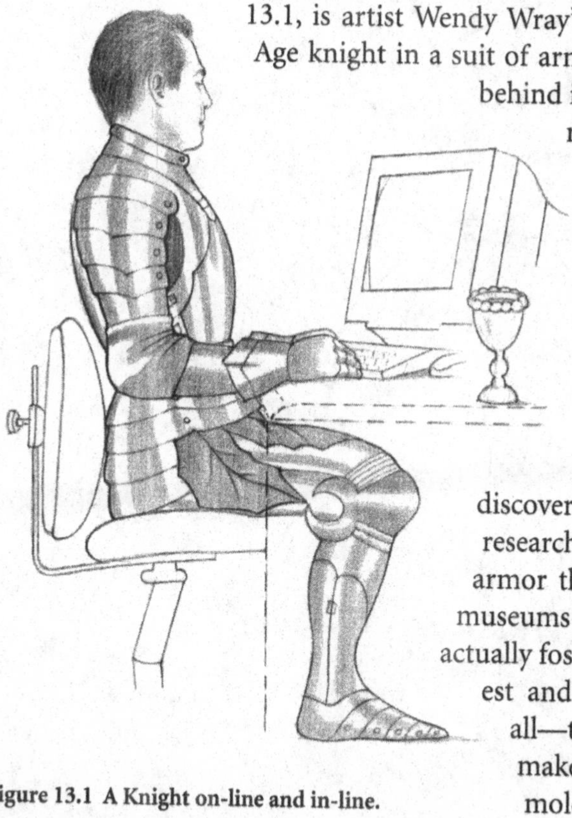

Figure 13.1 A Knight on-line and in-line.

the fully functional design of their customers: head high, shoulders back, spine curved, chest expanded, hips square. These "tin men" didn't come off a drawing board. What's visible on the outside is a product of what was once on the inside: muscles to bear lances and lanterns, bones to stand and deliver. The knight in shining armor was sculpted by days of fluid motion.

PCs don't need to be redesigned, nor do we. The design we were born with is right and ready for all seasons. It can take us from Camelot to cyberspace and beyond. Time's arrow stops only if we do. As always, the art of being—from being human to being digital—starts with being in motion. Look into the glittering surface of the armor, look into the past, and see the future—a future that doesn't have to hurt.

INDEX

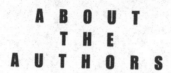

ABOUT THE AUTHORS

Pete Egoscue, an anatomical physiologist since 1978, operates the Egoscue Method Clinic in San Diego. His exercise therapy program is acclaimed worldwide for treating chronic musculoskeletal pain attributed to workplace and sports injuries, accidents, aging, and other conditions. He is also author with Roger Gittines of *Pain Free: A Revolutionary Method for Stopping Chronic Pain* and *The Egoscue Method of Health Through Motion.*

Roger Gittines is a writer living in Washington, D.C.